What they are saying about
Lower Your Cholesterol Without Drugs

I really didn't want to change my diet, give up my bad habits or start exercising. You've shown me a way to lower my cholesterol without taking drugs or changing my life. Now, I'm taking ten different supplements, not just for my high cholesterol, but for my general health.

—JOHN F., MIAMI, FL

I never knew there was any other way than prescription drugs. The drug I was on costs almost $100 a month, plus the doctor's visits and the liver tests they kept running on me. The supplements you said to take are very inexpensive, and I don't have to see the doctor all the time now. My cholesterol is much lower on these supplements than it was on the prescription I was taking.

—MARY L., PARMA, OH

I was overweight, ate the wrong foods, didn't take any supplements, and sat around watching TV for exercise. I stopped eating red meat, and butter and cheese for a start. I took some of the supplements in the book. I walk the dog every day now. I'm losing weight, and my cholesterol is now normal. This is really reasonable.

—PAUL J., LODI, CA

I had genetically high cholesterol and triglycerides, both over three hundred. The prescription drugs I took didn't lower them much at all, and they cost me a fortune! I had pretty much given up until I read your book. I take most of the supplements, and I changed my diet a lot. I joined the YMCA, and I swim three times a week now. My cholesterol and triglycerides are now in the high normal range, after only three months. I'm glad I discovered your book.

—CHARLES A., BOSTON, MA

Other Health Books
by Roger Mason

Lower Blood Pressure Without Drugs
The Minerals You Need
The Natural Diabetes Cure
The Natural Prostate Cure
No More Horse Estrogen!
The Supplements You Need
Testosterone Is Your Friend
What Is Beta Glucan?
Zen Macrobiotics for Americans

LOWER YOUR CHOLESTEROL WITHOUT DRUGS

A Practical Guide
to Using Diet and Supplements
for Healthy Cholesterol Levels

ROGER MASON

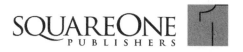

SQUAREONE
PUBLISHERS

Lower Cholesterol Without Drugs is not intended as medical advice. It is written solely for informational and educational purposes. Please consult a health professional should the need for one be indicated. Because there is always some risk involved, the author and publisher are not responsible for any adverse effects or consequences resulting from the use of any of the suggestions, preparations or methods described in this book. The publisher does not advocate the use of any particular diet or health program, but believes the information presented in this book should be available to the public.

All listed websites have been reviewed and updated during production. However, the data is subject to change.

COVER DESIGNER: Jeannie Tudor
EDITOR: Erica Shur
TYPESETTER: Gary A. Rosenberg

Square One Publishers
115 Herricks Road
Garden City Park, NY 11040
(516) 535-2010 • (877) 900-BOOK
www.squareonepublishers.com

Library of Congress Cataloging-in-Publication Data

Mason, Roger.
    Lower your cholesterol without drugs : curing high cholesterol naturally /
Roger Mason. — 2nd ed.
        p. cm.
    Rev. ed. of: Lower cholesterol without drugs / Roger Mason. © 2001.
    Includes index.
    ISBN 978-0-7570-0367-7 (pbk.)
  1. Low-cholesterol diet. 2. Anticholesteremic agents. 3. Dietary
supplements. I. Mason, Roger. Lower cholesterol without drugs. II. Title.
    RM237.75.M375   2012
    613.2'8432—dc23
                                                                    2011043286

Printed in the United States of America

10   9   8   7   6   5   4   3   2   1

Contents

Introduction

Coronary heart disease (CHD) is the main cause of death by far worldwide. The published international research on the effects of cholesterol and triglycerides on coronary heart disease is simply overwhelming and inarguable. *High blood fat levels are correlated with all-cause mortality (death from every major illness) and not just CHD!* Forty years of published international clinical research went into this book. There are many books available on heart and artery health, but nearly all of them are ineffective. This is not just a book on lowering blood fats, but one about total heart and artery health.

A low fat diet of natural foods is the only way to lower your blood fats. Your diet and lifestyle, not toxic drugs will provide you with a healthy heart. Statin drugs are the second most pre-scribed in America. Making better foods choices is the secret to a long and healthy life. Also, over forty natural supplements are discussed in detail. Beta-sitosterol, flax oil, beta glucan, and soy isoflavones are recommended as the cornerstone of your cho-lesterol supplement program. In no other book are you going to read an explanation of how your basic hormones affect your blood lipid levels. Diet, proven supplements, natural hormones, and exercise are the most important things you can do for a healthy heart and circulatory system.

Everyone who reads this book will have the ability to naturally improve their blood lipid profile, have better heart and artery health, and live longer, without resorting to taking drugs or surgery. *Prescription drugs only make you worse in the end.* Nature has answers for all our health conditions. You cannot poison your way to health.

Anyone can make continuing better choices in their daily food. You can choose an exercise you enjoy, even if it is just walking the dog a half hour a day. There are programs available to stop smoking, or drinking alcohol. It is easy to take the proven, inexpensive, effective, and safe natural supplements. You can balance your basic hormones cheaply, and without a doctor. These are things anyone can do.

I hope everyone who reads this book will put down their medication forever. *You don't need prescription drugs in your life.* You cannot poison your way to health. CHD is by far the biggest cause of death in the Western world. Don't be a statistic.

1. Cholesterol and Blood Diagnostics

Many of us hear about the dangers of high cholesterol on a daily basis, whether it's from health professionals in the media or from commercials hawking a low-cholesterol product. The simple fact is that high cholesterol kills, and the more you know about what it is, and whether or not you have it, the quicker you can act.

WHAT IS CHOLESTEROL?

Cholesterol is a soft, waxy substance that is found in your bloodstream and carried through your body in lipoprotein particles. It is made in your body and consumed in animal foods. We have fats (lipids) in our blood that are necessary for life. Vegans, who eat no cholesterol, still produce these with their livers. There are two types of cholesterol, high-density lipoprotein (HDL) and low-density lipoprotein (LDL). HDL is the good cholesterol. Its job is to collect, breakdown, and get rid of the LDL that may already be in your body. LDL is the bad cholesterol because it can form blockages from plaque build-up along your arteries and increase your risk of heart disease.

We are only going to be concerned with total cholesterol (TC), high-density cholesterol (HDL), low-density cholesterol

(LDL), triglycerides (TG), homocysteine (Hcy)—an amino acid produced by the body, uric acid (UA), and C-reactive protein (CRP)—a protein produced by the liver and found in the blood. Total cholesterol is the most important to measure. HDL takes cholesterol from the bloodstream into the liver, while LDL takes it back into the bloodstream. Therefore, we want high HDL and low LDL levels generally. Triglycerides are the form in which most fat is stored in the body; they are esters (stable forms) of fatty acids and glycerol. Obesity and diabetes are strongly correlated with high TG.

HOW IS CHOLESTEROL MEASURED?

When doctors draw blood to determine your cholesterol level, the laboratory performing the analysis measures the amount of cholesterol contained in a specific amount of blood. In the United States, cholesterol levels are measured in milligrams (mg) per deciliter (dl). In Canada, Europe, and Australia, it's measured in millimoles (mmol) per liter (L) of blood.

You should have your blood lipids measured annually as part of your medical checkup. The usual ceiling of 200 mg/dL (5.3 mmol/l) for total cholesterol is just too high—*150* mg/dL (3.95 mmol) is *the realistic ideal.* (Multiply the European number by 38 to get the American number.) Most rural, Asian people, and vegetarians, normally have levels of only about 150 mg/dL. This is a very practical and realistic goal. Divide your cholesterol level by your HDL level for the cholesterol-to-HDL ratio. For example, if your total cholesterol is 200 mg/dL and your HDL is 40 mg/dL (200 divided by 40) you have a ratio of 5.0. Men should be 4.0 or lower, and women should be 4.5 or lower. Triglycerides should be under 100 mg/dL (1.13 mmol.) (Multiply European by 88.3.) You can also use the home test kits available in the drug stores, but they only give values for total cholesterol.

Every year about 1.6 million Americans suffer heart attacks, and almost one-third of them die. The higher your cholesterol level, the more chance you have of not only having a heart attack, but suffering from stroke, atherosclerosis (clogged arteries), high blood pressure, Alzheimer's, cancer, diabetes, and overall early death. High cholesterol and triglycerides equal poor health and early death. *This cannot be debated.*

DANGERS OF HIGH CHOLESTEROL

The National Cholesterol Education Program has much to tell the public about the dangers of high cholesterol. Look at the following chart (*Archives of Internal Medicine* v 148, 1998) on cholesterol and death rates. A group of 361,662 men ages thirty-five to fifty-seven were studied for six years. The men with low cholesterol had only three deaths per 1,000 every year, while the men with high cholesterol had sixteen deaths per year. That is over 500 percent more fatalities. This is a huge difference, and clearly proves the diagnostic value of your total cholesterol

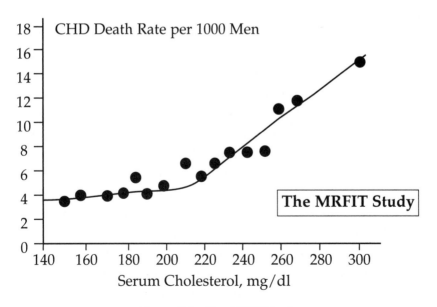

Figure 1.1   The MRFIT Study

level. *All-cause mortality, which is the combined reasons for death, is the gold standard.*

This Multiple Risk Factor Intervention Trial (MRFIT) study (see Figure 1.1), which was based on 361,662 men aged thirty-five to fifty-seven, was one of the largest, most important studies ever done on heart and artery health. The study has been covered in many medical journals due to the tremendous amount of information that was found. Here, you can see for yourself. Based on the studies of over a third of a million people, the lower your cholesterol (down to a level of about 150 mg/dL) the longer you are going to live. The higher your cholesterol, the less time you have on earth and the poorer your quality of life.

HOMOCYSTEINE LEVEL

It is very important you have your amino acid homocysteine (Hcy) level tested. The normal range is 5 to 15 mmol, so you must be in the lower range here and not merely midrange. A level that is under 10 mmol is good. Studies show that rural Mexicans with good diets, for example, had levels of 9, but urban Mexicans with westernized diets had levels of 12. A level over 15 is considered pathological (hyperhomocystemia). Levels over 15 cause *twice* the rate of CHD or coronary heart disease! The higher your Hcy level the more CHD of all kinds you will suffer from. Diet and life style are the right way to lower Hcy. Whole grains lower homocysteine. You can falsely lower this with a triple supplement of vitamin B-6 (2 mg), B-12 (as 1 mg methyl cobalamin), and folic acid (800 mcg), but this has not been shown to actually reduce CHD occurrence. In fact, at McMaster University, in Canada, 5,522 people were given this supplement for five years. Their homocysteine went down considerably, but there was no reduction in coronary heart disease. A better way to do this is taking 1,000 mg (2 x 500 mg) trimethyglycine (TMG) daily. The older you get, the higher your Hcy level goes. Men have higher levels than women.

Smoking, drinking coffee, high total cholesterol, and hypertension all raise Hcy. Diabetics, and those with insulin resistance, have higher levels. High Hcy is also associated with depression and dementia. Keep your level of Hcy under 10 micromoles with diet and life style.

C-REACTIVE PROTEIN LEVEL

It is very important to have your C-reactive protein (CRP) level tested. The hs-CRP (high sensitivity) test is an important inflammation marker. You want levels at 1.0 mg/liter or less on a 1.0 to 3.0 average range. CRP accurately predicts CHD conditions in general, as well as diabetes, and arthritis. High uric acid, hypertension, insulin resistance, smoking, high homocysteine, oral contraceptives, high total cholesterol, obesity, lack of exercise, and high triglycerides are major factors. You lower your CRP, as always, with diet and lifestyle. Less calories (not less food, but better food choices), more daily exercise, less fat (especially saturated fat), less animal protein (meat, dairy, poultry, eggs), less alcohol, weight loss, no smoking, a good mineral supplement, no birth control pills, no prescription drugs, and less sugar (any kind) intake are the ways to lower CRP. Weight loss and exercise stand out the most here. Rural Asians have very low CRP levels generally, due to low-fat diets and physical labor. Black Americans have higher levels generally. Again, exercise and weight loss are two effective ways to lower CRP.

URIC ACID LEVEL

It is also very important to have your uric acid (UA) level tested. Your level should be under 5.0 mg/dL for men and under 4.0 mg/dL for women. The conventional wisdom says that foods high in purines raise uric acid. A closer analysis shows this is not the real cause at all. Actually, *animal products per se raise uric acid levels.* Red meat of all kinds, poultry, eggs, milk and dairy products all raise your uric acid level. It's not just purines, since dairy products have almost no purines. The proof is that vegetarians, vegans, and macrobiotics have far lower uric acid in their blood. Americans who eat the most meat, due to their affluence, have the highest uric acid levels on earth. Most Asians, especially in China, Japan, Thailand, and Viet Nam, (who eat the least amount of animal products) have the lowest levels. Seafood in moderation does not raise uric acid. Sugars of all kinds also raise UA, and that includes honey, stevia, and fruit juice. *Sugar is sugar*!

High UA has been clearly correlated with hypertension, diabetes, insulin resistance, metabolic syndrome, low HDL, high LDL, high triglycerides, obesity, high insulin, high blood glucose, arterial plaque (clogged arteries), arterial stiffness, and coronary heart disease in general. At the Spokane Heart Institute, it was shown that people with levels over 5.2 mg/dL had 3.5 times the risk of cardiovascular death! The most stunning study of all was from the Radiation Effects Foundation in Japan (*Journal of Rheumatology* v 32, 2005). Here10,615 people were studied for a full twenty-five years. *A higher uric acid caused more all-cause mortality.* That means they died from every known cause! Men have higher levels than women. Women range from 2.4 to 6.0 mg/dL (average 4.2), so they should be under 4.0 mg/dL. Men range from 3.4 to 7.0 (average 5.2), so they should be under 5.0 mg/dL. Do not accept average levels here.

BLOOD SUGAR LEVEL

You should know your blood sugar level, and keep this under 85 mg/dL (5 mmol). (Multiply European by 17.) If you suspect any blood sugar problem, get an inexpensive one hour glucose tolerance test (GTT).This shows how your cells respond to insulin, and is much better than testing insulin itself. You want 20 points lower than the official suggested ideal level. High blood sugar and insulin resistance are predictive of coronary heart disease in general, as well as diabetes.

Urinary albumin excretion is also well correlated with coronary heart disease. This is called "microabluminurea." Also, get your creatinine checked if you get the uric acid test (UA). Both are excellent diagnostic tools for kidney health. Kidney disease is epidemic in America and closely related to heart and artery disease. This is mostly due to eating twice the protein we need.

CONCLUSION

They say an ounce of prevention is worth a pound of cure. The studies have shown that the first step towards helping yourself is to see where you stand. The tests we have discussed above will provide you with a measure of how high your risk factors are. Once you know, you can then take the easy-to-follow steps that you will find covered in the following chapters. By ignoring the potential dangers of a low level of HDL, and a high level of LDL, triglycerides (TG), homocysteine (Hcy), uric acid (UA), and C-reactive protein (CRP) in your bloodstream, you will be playing with fire. The next chapter will provide you with a look at just what these risks may entail.

2. Risks and Diseases

The published clinical evidence, over the last four decades, overwhelmingly shows that total cholesterol and triglycerides are the two most important diagnostic factors for overall cardiovascular health, quality of life, and longevity. Always remember, CHD is the biggest killer of all by far worldwide. A review of the published medical literature, for the past forty years, proves, beyond any doubt, that eating a diet high in saturated fats causes a rise in blood fats, and results in heart and artery disease. High fat diets, especially saturated animal fats, are a major cause of many other health problems such as diabetes, lung disease, kidney disease, pneumonia, Alzheimer's, and most all cancers. This massive evidence is based on millions of people, as well as epidemiological and migration studies. *This is simply inarguable.*

HIGH CHOLESTEROL AND HEART DISEASE

There are so many studies, it is almost impossible to choose which ones to use. We'll take the reviews and the largest studies. One review (*Atherosclerosis* v 118, 1995) from St. Bartholemew's Hospital in London looked at ten major cohort studies around the world. They said, "A systematic examination of the evidence on the relationship between serum cholesterol and ischaemic heart disease shows conclusively that serum cholesterol reduction, in populations with high rates of heart disease, is an effective and safe method of reducing heart disease rates." All of these very large studies proved that the higher the cholesterol levels, the more heart disease. No matter how much people lowered their levels (down to 150 mg/dL) there were continual beneficial effects. Again, we see that *the ideal is about 150 mg/dL.*

The MRFIT Study of 356,222 men leaves no doubt as to the facts. A chart from that study is on page 5, and shows the direct relation of cholesterol levels to heart and artery disease. This review (*Circulation* v 88, 1993) studied men from forty different countries. This showed that CHD rates rise as cholesterol levels go over 150 mg/dL. This is not just a phenomenon for people with higher levels over 200 mg/dL. For every 1 percent rise in your cholesterol level, you have a 2 percent rise in risk of coronary disease. The researchers said, "The relationship between serum cholesterol and six year risk of CHD death was continuous, graded, and strong over the entire range . . ." This means the ideal level is about 150 mg/dL, and anything over that raises your risk of CHD. They also found that, beyond any doubt, *diet was the major cause of high blood fats.* Dairy foods, such as milk and butterfat, were especially indicated.

The MRFIT study was also reviewed in the *Journal of the American Medical Association* (v 256, 1986). They said, "The relationship between serum cholesterol and CHD is NOT a threshold one, with increased risk confined to the two highest quintiles (groups divided into fifths), but rather is a continuously graded one that powerfully affects risk for the great majority of middle-aged American men." Again, this means that every point over a level of about 150 mg/dL greatly increases your chances of heart disease and early death.

The Seven Countries Study (*European Journal of Epidemiology* (v 9, 1993) had been ongoing for twenty-five years in 1993. Of all the factors they said, "Over 50 percent of the variance in CHD death rates in twenty-five years were accounted for by the difference in mean serum cholesterol." In Japan, men averaged approximately a level of 165 mg/dL total cholesterol; while in Finland, the Netherlands, and the United States, men had approximately a level of 250 mg/dL total cholesterol! As always, the lower the cholesterol level, the lower the coronary disease rate. Your cholesterol level is a far more important factor than smoking, drinking, exercise, or even blood pressure.

At Providence University, in Taiwan, (*Journal of the American College of Nutrition* (v 118, 1999) a study was done, with centenarians (people one hundred years of age and older), to see what factors allowed them to live so long. *Total cholesterol level was one of the very most important factors for predicting longevity.* Even though cholesterol levels are supposed to become less predictive as we age, this study showed that low blood lipids is always a central key to longevity, regardless of how old you are.

The American Heart Association published a Special Report in the journal *Circulation* (v 81, 1990) on the importance of cholesterol as the principal cause of CHD. "The evidence linking elevated serum cholesterol to CHD is overwhelming," they said. They reviewed all the major studies, especially the Framingham, Helsinki, and MRFIT since they are the largest in the world. To their credit, they said that diet is the most important factor, and the best solution to the problem, rather than drug treatment.

The famous Framingham Study again showed that total cholesterol, HDL, LDL, and triglycerides taken together are the single most important determinant of heart disease. We could go on quoting major studies like this, but the point is made, the proof is there, and there can be no doubts. Please look at Figure 2.1 on saturated fat consumption in forty countries and the death rate from heart and artery disease. *Saturated fat in your diet is the main cause of high blood fat levels.*

A twenty-five year follow-up was carried out on the Seven Countries Study (*Journal of the American Medical Asso-*

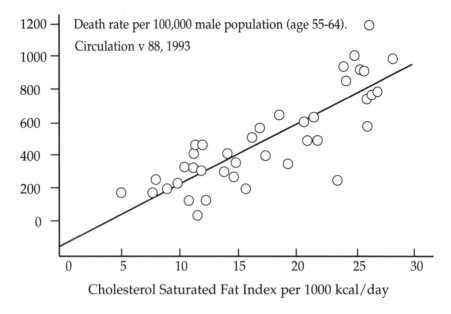

Figure 2.1. Cholesterol Saturated Fat Index per 1000 kcal/day
The more saturated fat you eat the more coronary heart disease you get based on 40 countries.

ciation v 274, 1995). In this research, 12,467 men in seven different countries were studied for ten years originally. "Across cultures, cholesterol is linearly related to CHD mortality, and the relative increase in CHD mortality rates with a given cholesterol increase is the same." They found cholesterol levels averaged 240 mg/dL for American men, 253 mg/dL for European men, but only 165 mg/dL for Japanese men (this was back in 1958, and the Japanese now average about 180 mg/dL). The Americans and Europeans had far higher CHD rates than the Japanese.

At the National Institute of Public Health in the Netherlands (*Netherlands Journal of Medicine* v 51, 1997), doctors found that cholesterol levels increased, in both men and women, as they aged. In both sexes, this increased *an astounding 60 points from the ages of about twenty-two to fifty-seven.* They said the main cause of this was clearly *the consumption of saturated animal fats.* They also agreed that many cohort studies have proven the correlation between serum cholesterol and mortality from heart disease. This risk is continuously graded with increasing levels. After the age of sixty, however, cholesterol levels tend to fall, due to poor health, and impaired liver function. These morbidly lowered results are misleading, since elderly people cannot make as much cholesterol.

Again at St.Bartholemew's Hospital (*European Journal of Clinical Nutrition* v 48, 1994) researchers looked at international studies. The results from seventeen different countries showed, "Variations in serum cholesterol accounted for 80 percent of the tenfold range of CHD across countries." *In other words, there was a ten times higher rate of illness and death in the higher levels, compared to the lower levels.* They also said, "These results show conclusively the efficacy and safety of attaining low cholesterol levels by dietary means in lowering the risk of CHD. Policies to achieve this objective should be a major public health strategy in the economically developed world." These medical doctors said that diet is the way to do this, and not reliance on drugs.

CONCLUSION

The published international research, over the last decade, have all come to the same conclusion. Total cholesterol, especially when used with triglyceride, homocysteine and C-reactive protein, is the best indicator we have for our risk of coronary heart disease—the largest killer by far in the developed world. Your LDL (low density cholesterol), and HDL (high density cholesterol) levels give an even bigger picture of your total heart and artery health. As you might expect, people with higher cholesterol and triglyceride levels also generally have higher CRP and homocysteine levels. These five parameters are central.

3. Diet, Diet, Diet . . .

A wholesome, low-fat, natural foods diet is the most important thing you can do to keep your blood fats at healthy levels. *Diet is the very key to health more than any other factor.* If you were eating well, you would not have a cholesterol problem. The supplements are very secondary to eating a low-fat diet that is high in whole grains and fiber. A diet based on whole grains, beans (all kinds), green and yellow vegetables, local fruits, soups, salads, and seafood (if you want), will allow you to live longer, and have a much higher quality of life. *Your fat calorie intake should only be 10 to 20 percent.* Any more than 20 percent just won't help you. Americans and Europeans eat over 40 percent fat calories, and most of these are saturated animal fats. *It is animal foods that cause high blood lipid levels.* Rural Asian people, of most all nationalities, traditionally have very low cholesterol levels. They eat very little animal fat. In their countries, the average cholesterol level is only about 150 mg/dL. The average American adult level is about 240 mg/dL. This is the main reason for our extreme CHD epidemic.

RED MEAT

Red meat such as beef, pork, and lamb, is the main cause of high blood fats. You don't have to be a vegetarian to change this, but you at least need to limit the amount of red meat you eat. You just can't eat one-half pound slabs of red meat every day and expect to have healthy cholesterol levels. If you insist on eating meat, get the most out of it by cutting a few ounces of lean meat into small pieces, marinating it, and stir-frying it with lots of vegetables. You can also use small amounts in soups. Fish and seafood are much better choices, if you aren't allergic. Fish and seafood, in moderation, do not raise your cholesterol or triglycerides. You don't need to eat meat! Take meat out of your diet.

POULTRY AND EGGS

Poultry and eggs are two of the top ten allergenic foods known. Many people have unknown allergies to both poultry and eggs; it doesn't matter whether the poultry is chicken, turkey, pheasant, duck, goose, or ostrich! Eggs are actually worse than poultry, because of the very high—i.e. 250 mg per egg—levels of cholesterol found in them. Take eggs out of your diet completely if you want to have healthy cholesterol levels. Using natural egg substitutes can be a *temporary* transition here.

DAIRY PRODUCTS

Low-fat dairy products are now widely available, but are still full of lactose and casein. *All adults of all races are lactose intolerant,* and no longer secrete the enzyme lactase. Casein is a proven cancer promoter that only exists in milk products. Lactose reduced dairy products do not solve the problem, nor do organically produced ones. Organic milk is a bad joke. This is discussed in the chapter on *Fats and Oils.* Use soy (or almond, oat, and rice) milk, soy cream cheese, soy yogurt, and soy cheese instead of dairy. These contain vegetable oils and no lactose. To see more on this go to www.notmilk.com, or www.milksucks .com. *Milk and milk products are the most allergenic foods on earth.*

WHOLE GRAINS

Whole grains should be the basis of your meals. Whole grains are literally the staff of life, and have been for centuries. Eat brown rice instead of white rice; eat whole wheat pasta instead of white pasta; eat whole grain bread instead of white enriched bread; eat whole grain cold cereals instead of the refined ones; eat more oatmeal, barley, buckwheat, and cornmeal. You can eat all the whole grains you want, never be hungry, and stay slim throughout your life. *Whole grains have been the staple food, of most civilizations, for the past five thousand years.* Countless studies prove the more whole grains you eat, the healthier you are and the longer you live.

VEGETABLES

Green and yellow vegetables come in a great variety. Learn to cook these fresh in a variety of cultural ways. Read cookbooks from around the world, and modify recipes as needed. Asians, generally, are the premier vegetable cooks. Some people think of vegetables as boring and lacking in taste, because they don't know how to cook them creatively. Vegetables contain many other important and necessary nutrients besides vitamins and minerals, such as sterols, lignans, antioxidants, and other vital constituents.

BEANS

Beans are considered by some as "peasant food," but beans should be a basic part of our diet. Pinto, black, northern, navy, garbanzo, pink, lentils, lima beans, kidney, cranberry, fava, aduki, red chili, and other beans make a wonderful addition to our diets. These are full of fiber, protein, vitamins, minerals, lignans, and other nutrients. Studies at universities, like Tulane and Arizona State, show that eating beans actually lowers our blood fats. The more beans and legumes you eat, the lower your cholesterol will be. Many published clinical studies have consistently shown beans help lower cholesterol and triglycerides.

FRUITS

Fruits, of course, have no fat or cholesterol, and should be eaten instead of sweetened desserts. Limit your fruit intake to about 10 percent of your diet. Sweeteners of all kinds, eaten in excess, will raise our blood fats. Sugar of any kind will raise triglycerides, due to disrupting our metabolism. Sugar is sugar is sugar. A study at the University of Minnesota (*American Journal of Clinical Nutrition* v 55, 1992) showed when healthy people were given modest amounts of common sugars such as fructose, this "resulted in significantly higher fasting serum total and LDL cholesterol, and also caused transient change in postprandial (after meals) serum lactate and triglycerides." Honey, maple syrup, molasses, agave, raw sugar, brown sugar, stevia, sucralose, evaporated cane juice, etc. are no better than regular white sugar. *All sweeteners are basically the same simple sugars*—sugar is sugar is sugar. Raw sugar is another bad joke. Fruit juice has just as much sugar as soft drinks, and this is mostly fructose. Yes, the same fructose you find in high fructose corn syrup.

If you don't want to be a vegetarian, seafood can be eaten in moderation. Fish and shellfish do not raise our cholesterol levels, are easily digested, and are very nutritious. A few people are allergic to fish and seafood. Nuts are generally 90 percent fat calories, and are only to be used as a garnish. It is best to avoid Nightshade family vegetables such as potatoes, tomatoes, eggplants, and all peppers. These contain toxic solanine. It is also good to avoid the most well known allergenic foods including citrus fruits, peanuts, yeast (bakers and brewers), chocolate, and coffee.

THE SCIENCE BEHIND A HEALTHY DIET

What scientific studies do we have that eating a low-fat, complex carbohydrate diet really works? Lots of studies, and we'll go over some of them briefly. At the Institute of Biomedical Science in Taiwan (*American Journal of Clinical Nutrition* v 58, 1993), young male and female vegetarians were studied. They ate diets of 63 percent whole complex carbohydrates. They had consistently lower cholesterol and triglyceride levels. Their other blood parameters such as uric acid, fibrinogen, and antithrombin were also excellent. You don't have to be a total vegetarian to gain these advantages in your health.

Another study, in the *American Journal of Clinical Nutrition* (v 83, 2006) was done at Harvard University. They stated very clearly, "Whole grain intake is inversely associated with risk of diabetes and ischemic heart disease in observational studies." They found the people who ate the most whole grains had lower cholesterol, lower triglycerides, lower blood sugar, lower homocysteine, lower C-reactive protein, and lower insulin levels. They concluded, "The results suggest a lower risk of diabetes and heart disease in persons who consume diets high in whole grains."

At the University of Otago, in New Zealand, (*European Journal of Clinical Nutrition* v 52, 1998), young (average age thirty-seven) healthy men were given either a traditional high-fat Western diet, or a low-fat diet based on complex carbohydrates from grains, vegetables, legumes, and fruit. The men on the healthy diet lost weight, their cholesterol levels fell, their HDL levels rose, while their LDL levels fell, all in only six weeks. They were allowed to select their own foods from a range of natural foods offered.

Another study, in the *European Journal of Nutrition* (v 55, 2001) was done on men and women in Norway. A group of 33,848 people (thirty-five to fifty-six years old) were studied for all cause mortality. Norwegians have a tradition of whole grain, especially bread, and eat far more than Americans. The more whole grains they ate, the less disease of all kinds they suffered from, and the longer they lived. They had lower cholesterol and lower blood pressure. They had fewer coronary heart disease and cancer deaths, as well as deaths from other causes. Whole grains equal a better and longer life.

A third study, in the *European Journal of Clinical Nutrition* (v 42, 2003), showed vegetarians have dramatically lower uric acid levels. It is important to maintain low uric acid levels. Eating animal foods, of all kinds, is the real cause of excessive uric acid. Some seafood, legumes, and other healthy foods have considerable purines, but do not raise uric acid. *High uric acid comes only from animal foods.* It is also a basic cause of kidney stones. Ten percent of Americans will eventually suffer from these stones.

At the University of Auckland (*Diabetes Research* v 63, 2004), people were allowed to eat all the low-fat natural food they wanted. They lowered their body weight, cholesterol, LDL, blood sugar, and blood pressure with no exercise or other changes. The more compliant they were, the more benefits they got. They simply made better food choices, and ate less fat.

Harvard University sponsored The Nurse's Study, and did a follow up for many years. The *Journal of the American Medical Association* (September 28, 2000) reported how many whole grains the 75,251 participants ate. The women who ate as little as two or three slices of whole wheat bread had up to 40 percent less ischemic strokes (the most common form) than the women who didn't eat whole grains. *The more whole grains they consumed, the less strokes they suffered from.* This study has been going on for over twenty years now. Strokes are the third leading cause of death in the U.S., and affect men and women equally.

The Physician's Health Study of 21,376 doctors (*Archives of Internal Medicine* v 167, 2007) found the more whole grain breakfast cereals the doctors ate the less heart disease, hypertension, stroke, diabetes and obesity they suffered from. "Our data demonstrate that a higher intake of whole grain breakfast cereals is associated with a lower risk of heart failure."

At the USDA Human Nutrition Center (*Journal of the American College of Nutrition* v 23, 3004), men with high cholesterol were fed a whole grain based diet, including brown rice, whole wheat, and barley. In just two weeks their total cholesterol fell 20 percent, their LDL fell 24 percent, triglycerides fell 16 percent, and HDL rose 18 percent. Studies like this show just how dramatically diet lowers blood fats with no other changes in lifestyle. Just adding proven supplements, exercise, and natural hormone balance would result in even more incredible results.

Dean Ornish (*Lancet* v 336, 1990) actually reversed clogged arteries in people in less than one year with a low-fat vegetarian diet. This is thought to be medically impossible. The patients were fed whole, natural foods with no other changes in their life styles. Dean does a lot of work in this area, and has written several books on natural diet.

CALORIE INTAKE

Not surprisingly, cholesterol and triglyceride levels are correlated with obesity. You can easily lose weight, without dieting, by simply *making better food choices.* You can literally eat more food with little calories when you choose better foods. You do not have to eat less food at all; you just have to eat healthier foods. You do not have to count calories, or adjust your portions either. The hunger drive is even more primal and more powerful than the sexual drive. No amount of willpower will stop you from eating when you're hungry. You must fill your stomach when you eat, and you can fill your stomach with delicious, low-calorie, natural food. You can enjoy your meals greatly, while staying slim and feeling good. Better food, not less food.

Calorie restriction is another important factor. *Americans eat twice the calories they need.* By making better food choices you eat less calories. Fats contain twice the calories of protein or carbohydrates. Eat two meals a day, rather than three. Don't snack. Fast one day a week on water from dinner to dinner. You will never be hungry doing these things, but can cut your calorie intake in half. *Eat more and weigh less.*

CONCLUSION

Billions of dollars are wasted every year treating the *symptoms* of obesity because we refuse to look at the *cause* of this overweight epidemic. Americans basically eat high-fat, low-bulk, low-fiber, high-calorie density, highly refined, high-sugar foods. We are overfed and undernourished. If you eat a high-fat diet, you will have high body fat. Vegetable oils are just as fattening as animal fats, and have the same amount of calories. You are what you eat, and the more fat you eat, the fatter you will be. A stick of butter has about 1,000 calories, but won't satisfy your hunger very well. In comparison, it would be impossible for most people to sit down and eat twenty apples, having the same 1,000 calories. A good book to read on how to eat all the delicious natural food you want, while staying healthy and slim with low blood fats is Terry Shintani's *The Hawaii Diet*. Other good books on eating well have been written by Dean Ornish, Neal Barnard, Susan Powter, Gary Null, Robert Pritikin, and any of the macrobiotic authors, such as Michio Kushi.

4. Fats and Oils

Saturated fats and cholesterol are basically found only in animal foods, *not in plant foods*. If you didn't eat red meat, poultry, eggs, and dairy products you wouldn't have a cholesterol problem in the first place. Yes, fish and seafood contain a little saturated fat and cholesterol, but, in moderation, do not raise your cholesterol or triglyceride levels. Most people are not willing to completely stop eating meat, poultry, eggs, and dairy. The ideal is not to eat these foods. It is certainly their right to eat them in *moderation*. However, it is simply impossible for you to eat these foods as staples and maintain healthy blood lipid profiles. A breakfast of bacon, eggs, and buttered toast is simply not reasonable. You can reduce the amount of animal foods in your diet and still be happy. You can certainly take the worst of these, like bacon, butter, and cheese, out of your diet and replace them with other foods. *Ideally, you want to eat 20 percent or less fat calories*, and mostly all calories should be from vegetable sources. The best diet for people recovering from heart or artery disease would only be 10 percent fat calories. Reducing your fat calorie intake to, say, 30 percent is just not going to show any benefits. *The magic number is 20 percent or less.*

DAIRY PRODUCTS

You may be looking at all those low-fat or no-fat dairy products out there, but they all contain lactose and casein. Lactose and casein are the problems with dairy, in addition to the saturated fat and cholesterol. What is wrong with milk sugar (lactose)? After the age of about three years old, all babies stop secreting the enzyme lactase, which digests the lactose. No adult of any race secretes lactase, and is therefore unable to digest milk sugar. Asians and Africans especially are sensitive to dairy products. Casein is proven to promote various cancers. *Milk is the number one allergenic food on earth.* There are a variety of very good tasting soy products you can replace dairy foods with. There are many brands of soy, rice, oat, and even almond milk. Lactose reduced milk is *not* the answer. Meltable, non-dairy cheese comes in a variety of traditional flavors such a cheddar, jack, parmesan, and mozzarella.

OILS

What oils are good for general use? Corn oil is good for general use, since it comes from grain. Safflower and sunflower oils are a good choice. Sesame is too expensive for general use. Olive oil is also a good choice. Soy oil does not taste good, unless it is so highly refined as to be nutritionless. Peanut oil comes from one of the top ten allergenic foods known, and should be avoided. Cottonseed oil was never meant for human consumption, and is merely sold for profit. It is a byproduct of the cotton industry. Walnut, avocado, almond, and other gourmet oils are expensive, and have limited use in salad dressings and such. Avoid anything that is labeled "vegetable oil," or "vegetable oil blend," as these can be almost anything! Usually it is cottonseed, or other cheap industrial oil in food grade. Palm and coconut oil are only for *occasional* use. These oils are really meant for the indigenous people in the hot, tropical areas where they are grown and produced. *All oils must be limited and used in moderation.*

Let's talk about canola oil. You see it endlessly promoted as healthy oil. This contradicts the facts completely. The name comes from "Canadian oil," and is from the rapeseed plant (from the Latin "rapa" or turnip). This contains less than 2 percent erucic acid. The normal rapeseed plant contains so much toxic erucic acid that humans and animals cannot eat the oil. The plant was extremely genetically engineered to lower its erucic acid content. Therefore, it cannot be called natural in any sense of the word. Avoid canola oil and any foods that contain it. It is purely a promotion for profit. The rapeseed plant was never meant by nature for human or animal consumption. *Avoid canola oil.*

CONCLUSION

Americans eat an astounding 42 percent fat calories, mostly saturated animal fats. Whole, natural foods supply all the essential fatty acids you need. You should take at least a gram (a mere 9 calories) or more of flax oil daily to supply omega-3 fatty acids. Eat as little fat in your diet as possible. It's fat that makes you fat, not food. Read the labels of every food you buy to see the percent of fat calories. Bake and broil your food, and stop frying it. Stop using fats like butter to flavor your food. You can eat all you want, when you eat healthy natural whole foods like whole grains, vegetables, beans, fruits, salads, and even seafood. You don't need to "go on a diet." *You just need* to *make better food choices.*

5. Trans Fatty Acids

Hydrogenated vegetable oils actually warrant a separate chapter for many reasons. These are the worst possible fats you can eat, and are even more harmful than the saturated animal fats. They are still in so many of our foods, and often well hidden, that it is difficult to avoid them. As of 2006, they must be separately listed on food labels if you get 0.5 g or more per serving. They are still put in many products! Hydrogenated oils do not exist in nature, so our bodies simply cannot recognize and digest them. People just don't realize how unhealthy these chemical abominations are, or they would quit eating them. Countless tons of these go into our food every year. Read the labels of everything you buy, and you'll be amazed at just how commonly found they still are. It is very difficult to avoid them in restaurants, since it is not required to list them on the menu.

Margarine is not, "better than butter," and never has been. Food manufacturers found they could extend the shelf life of foods, and make them less subject to rancidity, by using these toxic, cheap, artificial, man made creations. "Saturating" vegetable oils is done by subjecting inexpensive ones (like cottonseed and soy) to high pressure and heat, with hydrogen gas, using exotic catalysts like platinum. This extends shelf life at the cost of your health. In this chapter, we will prove to you beyond any doubt that these artificial laboratory creations are hurting your health and shortening your life. Never again knowingly buy or eat any foods containing them. There are many, many studies on the negative effects of trans fatty acids, but we will only look at a few of the most informative human ones done at some of the most prominent clinics. *Read your labels!*

THE SCIENCE BEHIND HYDROGENATED OILS AND SATURATED FATS IN OUR DIETS

At the University of Kuopio in Finland (*Metabolism Clinical & Experimental* v 48, 1999), healthy women were studied in a randomized, crossover protocol by giving them the usual highly saturated fat European diet, or diets high in hydrogenated oil. A mere 5 percent hydrogenated oil in their diet caused higher total cholesterol, LDL cholesterol, and triglyceride levels in just four weeks. They concluded that the hydrogenated fat diet "resulted in a higher total/ HDL cholesterol ratio, and an elevation in triglycerides and ApoB (a negative indicator for heart health) concentrations."

At Tufts University (*Metabolism Clinical & Experimental* v 45, 1996), elderly men and women were fed either a diet of 30 percent fat calories from corn oil, or one with hydrogenated corn oil margarine for a month. They then switched to the opposite diet for a month. The doctors found, "Mean total cholesterol levels were lowest when subjects consumed the corn oil diet as compared with the margarine diet." This is real world proof—with real people—that margarine raises your cholesterol levels, contributes to clogged arteries and heart disease, and causes poor quality of life, ending in early death.

At the National Public Health Institute in Finland (*American Journal of Clinical Nutrition* v 65, 1997), eighty healthy men were studied for their intake of trans fatty acids. Half the men were given diets high in saturated animal fats, and the other half were given diets equally high in trans fatty acids. They concluded that the diets that were high in trans fatty acids "had more adverse effects on lipoproteins than did equal amounts of animal fats." The intake of trans fats also worsened the LDL/HDL ratio. This is more proof that hydrogenated oils are much worse than saturated animal fats.

A lot of work was done at Wegeningen Agricultural University in the Netherlands. One group of researchers there (*Canadian Journal of Physiology* v 75, 1997) reviewed other major studies on the effects of trans fats on humans. They found that it is well established, "trans fatty acids raise serum LDL, and lower HDL in humans." They also found that trans fats raise lipoprotein A, "Lp(a)," which is a basic indicator of heart disease. They warned that, because of their adverse effects, all foods containing them should have clear statements on the labels as to the amounts therein. This was finally done in 2006. In another study there (*Journal of Lipid Research* v 33, 1992), healthy men and women were given diets based on either vegetable oil, animal fat, or hydrogenated oils. The researchers said, "7.7 percent of energy from trans fatty acids in the diet significantly lowered HDL cholesterol, and raised LDL cholesterol . . ." A third study at Wegeningen was another review of other major studies, with a full twenty-two references (*Current Opinion in Lipidology* v 7, 1996). The doctors came to the same conclusions as the others about the adverse effects of trans fatty acids in our diets. Europeans and Americans are eating about 5 to 15 grams a day, and the amount is rising. It should be zero grams a day. These should be completely banned from food.

A really impressive study was done with 748 men (*American Journal of Clinical Nutrition* v 56, 1992) at Brigham and Women's Hospital in Boston. This was a very in depth and complex study that measured many physiological parameters and biological markers. It was clear to the doctors that trans fats in our diets raise LDL levels, lower HDL levels, and raise total cholesterol. They said, "On the basis of results from other studies . . . this would correspond to a 27 percent increase in the risk of myocardial infarction (heart attack)." Trans fats in your diet, equal heart disease, and outright heart attacks.

Some more fine research was done at the University of Oslo in Norway (*Journal of Lipid Research* v 36, 1995), where young men were fed either margarine or butter in their diets. We've been told for many years now that, "margarine is better than butter," when, in fact, it is worse than butter. The men eating the margarine lowered their HDL levels. This just made their HDL/LDL ratio worse. The researchers concluded, "Consumption of partially hydrogenated oil may unfavorably affect lipid risk factors for coronary heart disease . . ." You don't need to use butter or margarine in your foods.

At the famous Harvard Medical School (Lancet v 341, 1993), doctors reviewed the very large and long term Nurses Study of 85,095 women, and how much margarine and hydrogenated oil they reported consuming. It was obvious that the intake of these fats was "directly related to risk of coronary heart disease," and that "consumption of partially hydrogenated vegetable oils may contribute to the occurrence of CHD." That's pretty clear.

Some very alarming work was done collaboratively at several clinics around the world, working together to study breast cancer (*Cancer Epidemiology Biomarkers Preview* v 6, 1997). They studied 698 cases of breast cancer in European women and concluded that, "The adipose concentration of trans fatty acids showed a positive correlation with breast cancer." This means they actually took biopsies (tissue samples) of breast tissue to analyze how much hydrogenated fats were actually in the bodies of the women from their dietary consumption. Now we have a proven link in humans showing the relation of eating unnatural trans fats to higher cancer rates.

At Limburg University in the Netherlands (*Journal of Lipid Research* v 33, 1992), doctors studied the effects of trans fats on levels of lipoprotein A, (also known as Lp(a)), which they called a strong risk factor for CHD. There were three strictly controlled experiments on healthy men and women who were fed saturated fats, monosaturated and polyunsaturated fats, or hydrogenated oils. The people on the hydrogenated oil diet raised their Lp(a) levels to very dangerous levels in only a month. They concluded, "These short-term experiments suggest that diets high in trans monosaturated fatty acids may increase serum levels of Lp(a)." If this was done in a month, imagine what the effects are after many years.

From time to time you will see studies in medical journals, such as a recent 2001 issue of the *Journal of the American Medical Association*. They will claim hydrogenated oils are very safe, or even preferable to natural fats and oils. Back to the old "margarine is better than butter" story. You will notice in small print in each of these so-called "studies," that they are funded and paid for by organizations such as the United Soybean Board and the National Association of Margarine Manufacturers. So much for objective science! Sorry to say, you can purchase space for your advertising, posing as science, in many medical journals today.

CONCLUSION

Folks, *read your labels*. Stop buying any foods that contain hydrogenated or partially-hydrogenated oils. Do not eat in fast food restaurants, as nearly everything they serve is full of these oils. You can find such things as potato chips and corn chips that aren't made with hydrogenated oils. You can occasionally use non-hydrogenated margarines such as Smart Balance®/Earth Balance® from your grocery store. You will be surprised at just how many foods contain these unnatural and dangerous synthetic oils. If a food has hydrogenated or partially-hydrogenated oils in it, don't buy it and don't eat it. *Read your labels!* When you eat out, ask the manager what kind of oil they use in the kitchen. Actually, trans fats should be completely banned.

6. Supplements

Making better food choices is the most important thing we can do for our health. Health is about diet and lifestyle. Supplements are important, but secondary to diet and a healthy lifestyle in lowering cholesterol and triglycerides, and improving CHD health. However, you receive far more health benefits from supplements and a proper diet, than with diet alone. All the supplements discussed in this chapter are natural, and safe. All the supplements mentioned are clinically proven effective supplements. They have clinical studies behind them to show their value. There are quite a number of supplements, and you will find these supplements presented in alphabetical order.

SUPPLEMENTS FOR LOWERING YOUR CHOLESTEROL

Acetyl-l-carnitine

Acettyl-l-carnitine (ALC) is a much more effective form of L-carnitine. This is also very important for brain metabolism, and maintaining good memory and clarity of thought as you age. All the studies on L-carnitine would be even more effective with ALC. This is a very important supplement for everyone over the age of forty.

Dosage: Take 500 to 1,000 mg a day.

Acidophilus

Acidophilus is important in order to keep our intestinal flora (good bacteria that digest our food) in balance, and prevent growth of the harmful bacteria. Our large intestine digests all fats. This is where cholesterol is either absorbed or excreted. Various studies have shown that acidophilus is also good for cardiovascular health. Poor digestion is an epidemic, due to eating too much food, refined foods, too much fat, too much protein, drinking coffee and alcohol, and eating too much sugar. Be sure to take FOS and L-glutamine with your acidophilus for best effect. *Strong digestion is the heart of good health.*

Dosage: Purchase a good refrigerated brand, with at least 6 billion units per capsule containing six to eight different strains, and keep it refrigerated.

Alginate

Alginate (sodium alginate) is an effective, natural seaweed extract. It is very effective for lowering blood lipids, and removing toxic heavy metals like mercury, lead, and cadmium from our blood. Scientists have known about these benefits for decades now, but it never became a popular supplement for some reason. It is not easy to find this at the retail level, so just Google "sodium alginate." This is an inexpensive, safe, and an overlooked way to lower your cholesterol. *Alginate is safe, inexpensive, proven, and effective.*

Dosage: Take about three grams a day for one year, as it is exogenous.

Beta Carotene

Beta carotene is a good antioxidant to take, and will work with other supplements synergistically to lower cholesterol. This is a better choice than taking vitamin A, and has many other benefits for your health generally. There are many studies on beta carotene showing how powerful and effective it is as an antioxidant, how it helps regulate cholesterol metabolism, and protects against atherosclerosis. This should be a part of your daily supplement program for many other reasons than just lowering cholesterol.

Dosage: Take 10,000 IU daily of any good brand.

Beta Glucan

Beta Glucan is discussed in Chapter 10.

Beta Sitosterol

Beta Sitosterol is discussed in Chapter 8.

Carnosine

Carnosine (L-carnosine) is an amino acid that helps support good heart health. It reduces glycation (sugars binding to proteins) and has anti-aging properties. It is found in our muscles basically. There is good science behind carnosine. Since CHD is the biggest killer by far, this is important for anyone over forty. Anyone concerned about their heart and artery health should take this. This should be a definite part of your supplement program.

Dosage: Take 500 to 1,000 mg a day.

CoQ10

CoQ10 is a very heart healthy supplement. Buy real Japanese uniquinone, and not ubiquinol. Ubiquinol has no stability. All "special delivery systems" are merely promotional claims. Levels fall as we age, and this is not found in food. This is a very important supplement for anyone over the age of forty. This is very important for total cardiovascular health.

Dosage: Take 100 mg and no less. Take your CoQ10 with food or flax oil for best absorption.

Curcumin

Curcumin is the active ingredient in the spice tumeric. This has been used in Indian Ayurvedic medicine for over 1,000 years. There are lots of good studies on using curcumin for lowering cholesterol. This is temporary and exogenous, so only take it for six to twelve months. This is completely optional.

Dosage: Take at least 500 mg of actual curcumin, as stated on the label.

Vitamin C

Vitamin C is a fine antioxidant when used in moderation of 250 mg or less a day. Taking megadoses acidifies our naturally alkaline blood and unbalances our system. Long term studies show the dangers of using megadoses. Claims are made that taking several grams a days (3,000 to 5,000 mg) will result in great health benefits. *None of these are true.* Studies prove that taking such doses result in much more debilitating side effects than benefits. Do not overdose on this or any other supplement.

Dosage: We only need about 60 mg. Limit this to 250 mg a day.

Vitamin D

Vitamin D cannot be emphasized enough. This is actually a powerful oil soluble hormone. This is not found in your food, and most people do not get out in the sun enough to synthesize it. Deficiency of vitamin D is epidemic, especially as we age. Avoid overdoses as this is fat soluble.

Dosage: Be sure to take the 400 IU in your daily vitamin supplement, as well as an extra 400 IU (unless you are out in the sun regularly). Limit your intake to 1,200 IU if you are not out in the sun. Do not take more than this. Dark skinned people may be vitamin D resistant however, and need more.

DIM

DIM (di-indolylmethane) is important to help keep estradiol and estrone levels low. High estrogens in men or women are harmful to our overall health. All "special delivery systems" are simply promotional claims.

Dosage: Take 200 mg with flax oil or food.

Vitamin E

Vitamin E is important for heart and artery health. Forty years ago the medical world would not even admit vitamin E was a necessary nutrient! This is found in whole grains, and it is very deficient in our diets. We only eat one percent whole grains! The studies on vitamin E and CHD health go back forty years, and they are overwhelming. This is definitely one of the basic supplements you want to take daily. Your multivitamin will most probably only contain the RDA of 30 IU.

Dosage: Take 200 IU of any good brand you like (or 400 IU every other day), but be sure to choose the natural, mixed tocopherols, not synthetic d-alpha. People with heart problems can take 400 IU. This amount, 400 IU, will tend to thin your blood.

Fibers

Fibers generally, especially psyllium, are very good for keeping your cholesterol low, and they will also help keep your bowel movements regular. You can use sea fiber like chitin, or the usual plant fibers like guar gum, glucomannon, fruit (apple or citrus) pectin, oat bran, wheat bran, or others. Ideally your diet should be full of fibers, especially from whole grains and various beans.

Dosage: Eating a naturally high fiber diet is the best way to get your daily fiber intake rather than taking a supplemental form.

Flax Oil

Flax oil is discussed in Chapter 9.

FOS

FOS is short for fructooligosaccharides, otherwise known as insulin. It is an extract of chicory root. This supplement has been around for a long time, but only recently was it discovered that this feeds your good intestinal bacteria. The higher your levels of beneficial flora in your intestines, the lower your cholesterol levels generally. FOS is very good for your intestinal health, and has good science behind it. Anyone with intestinal disorders should consider using this in larger doses (like 1.5 grams twice a day) for a year. Abstinence from alcohol and coffee, a low-fat—low sugar—high fiber diet, and eating lower calorie whole foods will improve your digestion greatly.

Dosage: FOS is widely available, and you should take one or two 750 mg capsules a day with your acidophilus. Take FOS along with a refrigerated brand of acidophilus and some L-glutamine every day.

Garlic

Garlic has many proven health benefits. Human studies over the years have verified the advantage of garlic supplements for better cholesterol levels. Just buy pint (or quart) jars of chopped garlic, and cook with it.

Dosage: It is important to get a good, reliable brand with high levels of active ingredients stated on the label. Use fresh garlic in your daily cooking.

Glucomannon

Glucomannon is a plant fiber from the konjac root; it may help you eat less, while lowering your cholesterol. It is inexpensive and widely available. It swells up in your stomach giving you a feeling of fullness. This may cause you to eat less, and still feel full. There are many studies, including human ones, on the effectiveness of glucomannon.

Dosage: You should take at least 2 to 3 grams a day prior to meals. Take this for just one year.

Glucosamine

Glucosamine is very important for bone health. This needs co-factors such as calcium, magnesium, boron, silicon, and vitamin D. It also needs hormone support, especially from testosterone, DHEA, progesterone and estriol (in women). Ninety-five percent of Americans over sixty-five are arthritic. Glucosamine does not work alone. Chondroitin has no published human clinical research to verify the claims made for it.

Dosage: Take 500 to 1,000 mg of glucosamine a day. Remember that glucosamine needs cofactors to be effective.

Glutamine

Glutamine is a common amino acid known as L-glutamine. This is a proven inexpensive supplement. L-glutamine has shown very impressive benefits for intestinal health. Progressive surgeons are giving it to their patients after intestinal surgery. It also has been shown to spike levels of human growth hormone when taken in doses of one gram two times a day (AM and PM). The scientific literature has recently published many studies on the benefits of L-glutamine supplementation. This is a definite part of your supplement program, and will help keep your intestines full of good bacteria and free of the bad bacteria.

Dosage: You should take at least 2,000 mg (four 500 mg tablets) of L-glutamine a day (two tablets in the AM and two tablets in the PM). You can buy bulk glutamine, and take one to two tablespoons a day.

Glutathione

Glutathione is one of the two basic antioxidant enzymes that help fight dangerous free radicals, and are involved in cholesterol metabolism. Ironically, taking oral glutathione does a poor job of raising blood levels. Fortunately, there is a supplement called N-acetyl-cysteine, or "NAC," that effectively raises glutathione levels. Unfortunately, the other basic antioxidant enzyme, SOD (superoxide dismutase), is not absorbed orally. This must be injected or used in a nasal spray to be absorbed. Doctors do not have injectable SOD yet. NAC is a good general supplement for anyone over the age of forty.

Dosage: Take a 600 mg NAC capsule daily.

Grape Seed Extract

Grape seed extract is a temporary, exogenous supplement. Grape *skin* extract is known as resveratrol, and there is just no good, published, human independent clinical science behind it.

Dosage: Take for only one year or less.

Guar gum

Guar gum is a very good fiber to use. It is easier to take in capsules. Mixing this with any liquid will thicken it up so much it will be hard to drink. It is commonly used in small amounts as a thickener in foods such as salad dressing. There are many studies on the benefits of this fine fiber. It comes from the Cyamopsis plant in India. Surprisingly, there are lots of studies on this natural supplement. It is inexpensive and widely sold.

Dosage: Like other such fibers, you need at least two to three grams a day for results. Take for only one year, as this is exogenous.

Guggul Gum

Guggul Gum is a fine exogenous supplement you can take for six to twelve months. Not only does this help lower cholesterol, lower triglycerides, raise HDL and lower LDL, but also lowers uric acid. Human studies have shown up to a 15 percent drop in total cholesterol, and a whopping 26 percent in triglycerides with no change in diet or exercise. Not everyone will get such dramatic results however. Admittedly, there is not a lot of published human clinical science.

Dosage: Take 250 mg of 10 percent extract so that you get 25 mg of actual guggul sterones. This may be taken for six to twelve months.

Lecithin

Lecithin emulsifies dietary fats so they can be digested more easily. It works by decreasing the absorption of cholesterol in our intestines, and by other mechanisms. This soybean extract is sold everywhere and is very inexpensive. It is also known as phosphatidyl choline, and is good for brain health, memory, and liver function. (Do not confuse it with "PS" or phosphatidyl serine, which is also a fine supplement for brain health in 100 mg doses.) This is a good choice for good heart and artery health, with studies going back for many years. Lecithin has been shown to lower total cholesterol, LDL cholesterol, and homocysteine levels, as well as being antiatherogenic and helping keep our arteries clear of fat buildup.

Dosage: Take a 1,200 mg softgel daily.

Lipoic acid

Lipoic acid blood levels fall as we age. This is not found in your food. *R-only lipoic acid is completely unnecessary and overpriced.* High blood sugar is strongly associated with coronary heart ailments, as is insulin resistance. Keep your blood sugar under 85 mg/dL. High blood sugar is an epidemic.

Dosage: Take 400 mg of regular R,S-lipoic acid to maintain low blood sugar levels.

Magnesium

Magnesium is a vital mineral that deserves separate mention since it has many proven benefits. Magnesium should definitely be a part of your supplement program, as calcium cannot be absorbed, without magnesium, boron, strontium, and silicon. There are numerous scientific studies on magnesium supplements that show various benefits to health. This includes lower cholesterol and even lower blood pressure. Make sure your mineral supplement contains this. Magnesium does not work alone, and must have all the other basic nineteen minerals with it.

Dosage: Even if you are eating a diet rich in whole grains (the best source), it is still wise to take about 250 mg daily.

Minerals

Minerals are very important to every aspect of our health. The importance of getting all the minerals and trace elements we need for proper cholesterol synthesis and metabolism is not generally recognized. We are all mineral deficient in some way. Mineral deficiency is linked to every health condition known. You need at least twenty elements, including calcium, magnesium, iron, zinc, boron, selenium, chromium, iodine, molybdenum, manganese, copper, germanium, strontium, nickel, tin, cobalt, gallium, cesium, silicon, and vanadium. More research needs to be done in this area. Search the internet under "mineral supplements" to find a comprehensive one that includes most or all of the elements we have discussed in this chapter. Read the label to make sure the *amount* of each mineral is clearly stated. *Read the label.*

Dosage: To learn the optimal daily intake for each of these vital minerals, refer to Table 6.1 on pages 50 and 51. This table provides you with the appropriate doses of all twenty minerals. Minerals are covered in detail in Chapter 7: The Minerals You Need.

Niacin

Niacin, niacinamide, and "non-flushing" niacin overdoses are NOT good choices for lowering your cholesterol, regardless of the hype you've read. An overdose of any supplement unbalances your metabolism, even watersoluble vitamins. Always remember that megadoses of anything unbalance your body and hurt your health.

Dosage: You only need 20 mg a day.

Phosphatidyl Serine

Phosphatidyl serine (PS) is an important supplement to take for brain health. This works well with ALC and pregnenolone. This is a well proven supplement for cognition, memory, clarity of thought, and to prevent senility.

Dosage: Take 100 mg a day.

Policosanol

Policosanol (aka octacosanol) is promoted for lowering cholesterol. However, all the "studies" come from a unrecognized clinic in Cuba. There is simply no valid published human science here. Stick to clinically proven supplements.

Pectin

Pectin is found basically in the inner rind of citrus fruits, and in apples. All are inexpensive and very effective. *Modified pectin is very expensive, and offers no advantages at all.* Plain old, regular, inexpensive citrus or apple pectin is a very effective and readily absorbable fiber. There is good science behind all pectins. There are other health benefits to taking pectin. Take for one year. It is a good, safe, proven, effective, but exogenous supplement.

Dosage: Like the other fibers, you need to take at least 2 to 3 grams daily. Take only for one year.

Red Rice Yeast

Red rice yeast has been promoted for lowering cholesterol. There is almost no valid science here, and it hasn't been proven to be safe. Supposedly this contains a "natural version" of a statin drug. A study at East Tennessee State University showed it was, in fact, toxic. This is reason enough not to use it.

SOD

Sod (superoxide dismutase) is the second antioxidant enzyme. Our levels fall as we age, and low SOD levels have been consistently correlated with high blood lipids. The problem is that there are no practical SOD supplements. It must be injected or used intranasally, and doctors do not have SOD, or even know about it. It is not legal to prescribe it sublingually or as a nasal spray. *The oral SOD tablets sold have no value.* Real SOD is biosynthesized and costs one-thousand dollars a pint. You can find topical SOD creams, but these are not transdermal, and won't raise your blood levels. Hopefully this will become available in the future.

Soy Isoflavones

Soy isofavones are discussed in Chapter 11.

Spirulina

Spirulina has been hyped for a long time now as some kind of wonder food. It is simply fresh water algae, as is chorella. There are no valid studies in the last forty years on any benefits from taking spirulina, much less to lower blood fats, and no active ingredients were ever identified.

Taurine

Taurine is a common amino acid that can be used temporarily to help lower our blood fats. There are also benefits for diabetes and other blood sugar conditions. This is a temporary supplement.

Dosage: Take 500 mg for one year, even though it is endogenous and found in our daily food and in our bodies.

Tea

Tea (green) really does work, and will help your cholesterol levels. The catechins and polyphenols found in green tea are very powerful antioxidants. Find a *decaffeinated* brand and do not take the inexpensive brands that are full of caffeine. This is simply common black tea before it is fermented. Many studies have been done on the health benefits generally, and the active ingredients. It is bothersome that it is naturally full of caffeine. This is completely optional.

Dosage: Take this for only one year, as it is exogenous and not a common food.

TMG

TMG (also known as trimethylglycine and betaine) has powerful rejuvenation properties for our liver. The human studies on this are most impressive. Our livers are stressed from our high-fat diets, use of prescription drugs, recreational drugs, alcohol, coffee, and preservatives. The liver is our largest internal organ, and processes the fats in our blood. *The liver and gall bladder are central to cholesterol metabolism.* This is very important to do! Take TMG to rejuvenate and cleanse your liver.

Dosage: Take 3 grams of this every day for six to twelve months to cleanse and strengthen your liver. After a year, take 1 gram (2 X 500 mg) a day for maintenance and lower Hcy levels.

Vitamins

Vitamins only number thirteen, and there is an RDA for each of them. You can easily find a complete vitamin formula with all thirteen in the recommended RDAs. Find a brand with 1 mg of methyl cobalamin, instead of regular B-12. Do not buy any that use regular B-12, as it simply doesn't absorb. Regular vitamin B-12 must be injected.

Dosage: The list of vitamins and the optimal daily dosage are in Table 6.1 on pages 49 and 50.

OTHER SUPPLEMENTS TO CONSIDER

If you are over forty, or have a medical condition of some kind, there are temporary, exogenous (not in your body or your food) supplements you can also take for six to twelve months for your general health. Quercetin (100 mg) is a strong antioxidant found in apples and onions, and well worth taking. Aloe vera gel (200:1 extract) is a fine, traditional temporary supplement. Take two 100 mg capsules. Milk thistle extract (two capsules) is another temporary supplement that can be used to cleanse and tone your liver. Ellagic acid from walnut hulls (100 mg) is a temporary supplement that has shown anti-cancer and other properties.

We now have children with high cholesterol and triglycerides, for the first time in human history. Children, teenagers, and people under forty, don't need many supplements. They can take beta glucan, flax oil, acidophilus, FOS, L-glutamine, a good mineral supplement, a good vitamin supplement, vitamin D, and vitamin E. An eighty-pound child would need half doses, and a forty-pound child will need quarter doses. This would apply as well for your pets; a twenty-pound dog would only need eighth doses.

Popular supplements such as lycopene, chondroitin, nattokinase, noni juice, colloidal minerals, sea silver, colloidal silver, coral calcium, hoodia cactus, resveratrol, 5-HTP, deer antler, modified citrus pectin, astaxanthin, saw palmetto, Pygeum africanum, maca root, chrysin, MGN-3, AHCC, whey protein, oral SOD, megadoses of *anything*, Gymnema sylvestre, MSM, 7-keto DHEA, evening primrose oil, horny goat weed, tongkat ali, tribulis terrestis, coconut oil, bilberry, pomegranate products, arginine, cat's claw, brewer's yeast, shark cartilage, ginger root (for arthritis), oral hyaluronic acid, cranberry juice capsules, DMAE, CLA, goji berries, OTC (over-the-counter) growth hormone secretagogues, OTC testosterone boosters, acai fruit, mangosteen products, *any weight loss product, any* sexual rejuvenation formula, all bee products, all homeopathic products, and other such items simply have no valid, independent, published human research. Just take the ones with international published clinical studies to validate them.

AN OVERVIEW OF IMPORTANT DAILY SUPPLEMENTS

The table below lists the most important supplements you should take on a permanent basis in order to help lower your cholesterol and to maintain good health in general. Beside the name of each supplement, you'll find the optimal daily intake, which is not necessarily the same as the reference daily intake (RDI) established by the Food and Drug Administration (FDA). Note, for example, that the RDI for vitamin E is only 30 IU, but the *optimal* daily intake is 200 IU.

TABLE 6.1. PERMANENT DAILY SUPPLEMENTS		
Supplements	Optimal Daily Intake	Considerations
VITAMINS		
Vitamin B_1 (Thiamine)	1.5 mg	
Vitamin B_2 (Riboflavin)	1.75 mg	
Vitamin B_3 (Niacin)	20 mg	
Vitamin B_6	2 mg	
Vitamin B_{12}	2 mg	
Vitamin C	60 mg	Do not take more than 250 mg in one day.
Vitamin D	800 IU	If you are sick or elderly, take up to 1,200 IU a day.

Supplements	Optimal Daily Intake	Considerations
VITAMINS (cont.)		
Vitamin E	200 IU of mixed natural tocopherols	Or take 400 IU every other day.
Vitamin K	80 mcg	
Biotin	300 mcg	
Folate (Folic Acid)	400 mcg	
Pantothenic Acid	10 mg	
MINERALS		
Boron	3 mg	
Calcium	250 mg	Some suggest taking 1,000 mg of calcium a day, but only dairy intake will give you this much calcium and it is better to avoid eating dairy.
Cesium	100 mcg	
Chromium	120 mcg	
Cobalt	100 mcg	
Copper	2 mg	
Gallium	100 mcg	
Germanium	100 mcg	
Iodine	150 mcg	
Iron	10 mg for men, 18 mg for women	
Magnesium	400 mg	
Manganese	2 mg	
Molybdenum	75 mcg	
Nickel	100 mcg	
Selenium	70 mcg	
Silicon	10 mg	
Strontium	1 mg	

Supplements	Optimal Daily Intake	Considerations
MINERALS (cont.)		
Tin	100 mcg	
Vanadium	1 mg	
Zinc	15 mg	
OTHER NUTRIENTS		
Acidophilus	6 billion live multi-strain organism capsules	Buy and keep refrigerated. Take once or twice daily.
Acetyl-L-carnitine	500 to 1,000 mg	
Beta-carotene	10,000 IU	
Beta Glucan	200 mg or more	
Beta-sitosterol Complex	300 to 600 mg	
Coenzyme Q_{10}	100 mg	If you are ill, take 200 mg daily for one year. Take with food, or flax oil as Coenzyme Q_{10} is oil-soluble.
Di-indolyl Methane (DIM)	200 mg	Take with food, or flax oil as DIM is oil-soluble.
Flaxseed Oil	1,000 to 2,000 mg	Buy and keep refrigerated. Take once or twice daily.
Fructo-oligo-saccharides (FOS)	750 to 1,500 mg	
Glucosamine	500 to 1,000 mg	
L-glutamine	2,000 mg	Take two 500 mg tablets in the a.m. and two in the p.m.
Lipoic Acid	400 mg	
N-acetyl Cysteine (Glutathione)	600 mg	
Phosphatidyl Serine (PS)	100 mg	
Quercetin	100 mg	
Soy Isoflavones	40 mg of daidzein and genistein	If you drink soy milk regularly, you probably don't need this.

CONCLUSION

Too often our diets lack the proper nutrients. Yet with so many different nutrients available on the market, it is difficult to determine which ones you actually need. By understanding the role the nutrients discussed in this chapter play in maintaining good health, along with a naturally healthy diet and lifestyle, you can better understand how they can work effectively toward lowering your cholesterol and maintaining general good health. However as you will see in the following chapters, there are other important elements to consider in creating a comprehensive program for yourself.

7. The Minerals You Need

Studies have shown us how important minerals are to our health. Good mineral nutrition helps us to live longer, healthier lives. There are only ninety-one natural elements. Taking out the gases, halogens, sulfur, phosphorous, sodium, potassium, and carbon leaves seventy-three possible elements needed for human and mammalian nutrition. Science has shown how important minerals are for any disease or medical condition. *Every single health problem known is due in part to mineral deficiency.*

MINERALS TO LOWER YOUR CHOLESTEROL

We're all mineral deficient—no matter how well we eat. There are only ten elements officially classified as essential, with a set RDA. There are at least twenty-four elements we need. We get sufficient sulfur, potassium, phosphorous, and sodium in our daily diet. The best mineral supplements sold generally only contain about ten elements. Search the internet under "mineral supplements" to find a comprehensive one that includes most or all of the ones discussed in this chapter. Read the label, and look at the amounts contained in the product. Colloidal minerals, coral calcium, and the like do not state how much of each on the label, as they contain no significant biological amounts.

CALCIUM

Calcium is the most abundant element in our bodies, and 9 percent is found in our bones. It is essential, of course, but the RDA of 1,000 mg is simply not scientifically sound at all. Only dairy products contain large amounts of calcium, and you shouldn't be eating any milk products There is little problem with calcium intake; *the real issue is absorption.* There is just too much emphasis and research on calcium, and not enough on the other vital elements.

Dosage: A reasonable figure would be 400 mg a day. Calcium needs cofactors, such as magnesium, boron, strontium, silicon, omega-3s, and vitamin D in order to be absorbed and make bone. It also needs hormonal factors such as testosterone, DHEA, progesterone, and estriol (in women).

MAGNESIUM

Magnesium is the fourth most abundant element in our bodies, with an RDA of 400 mg. Deficiency is common, since Americans only eat about 300 mg. Common salts are good. *The main source is whole grains,* but we only eat about 1 percent whole grains now. Magnesium is the center of the chlorophyll molecule, which is the life blood of the plant world. There is massive research on magnesium, and this is a very heart healthy mineral. Eat lots of whole grains.

Dosage: Take a supplement of 200 mg to 250 mg a day.

IRON

Iron is one of the ten essential elements, and deficiency is as common as ever. Even with our excessive consumption of red meat and animal products (the most abundant source), many people just don't absorb what they need. Copper is needed for absorption, and there is an important iron-to-copper ratio. Iron is occasionally found in high levels in hypercholesterol conditions, but this is due to an excretion problem, and *not excessive intake.* Iron retention, and lack of excretion, fortunately is a rather rare problem. Iron is the "heme" in hemoglobin, and the basic mineral in our blood. Iron is the center of our red blood cells, and this is why it is so important. You shouldn't be eating red meat, so you won't have to worry about overconsumption.

Dosage: A good supplement will contain the female RDA of 18 mg. The male RDA is only 10 mg. Common sulfates, fumarates, and gluconates are good.

ZINC

Zinc is one of the ten essential elements. Most of the zinc in the male body is found in the prostate gland. Blood levels may be either high or low in those with high blood fats; there is just no consistency here. There is an important zinc-to-copper balance. Zinc is found in whole grains, beans, nuts, and meats. Deficiency is especially common in the poor, elderly, and alcoholics. There are about 2.5 g of zinc in the human body, almost half of which is in the muscles. Whole grains and beans are the best source.

Dosage: Most people need 15 mg RDA. Never take in more than 50 mg of zinc daily, as the toxicity level is low. The usual citrates, oxides, and sulfates all work well.

BORON

Boron is definitely *the most deficient mineral in our diet.* It wasn't until 1990 that boron was even accepted as essential! The research is overwhelming here. Our soils and food are very boron deficient. You would think that all vitamin and mineral supplements would contain 3 mg of this inexpensive and vital element, but very few do. This proves the megacorporations have huge advertising budgets, but no research departments. Americans, probably, only take in a mere 1 mg a day. Be sure you get this in your supplement, as boron deficiency is all too common. There is great science behind boron.

Dosage: There is no official RDA, but 3 mg is the suggested daily intake. Citrates or common boric acid is fine here.

MANGANESE

Manganese is essential. There are a mere 20 mg in the average human body. Whole grains are a major source, along with beans and legumes, nuts, and root vegetables. Most people do get enough, especially vegetarians. There is an abundance of research showing the benefits for our health. A supplement is still good insurance for such an important element. This is found in most mineral supplements. There are too many uses to list, but arthritis and bone problems are important areas of study.

Dosage: The RDA was only recently established at 2 mg. Sulfates and oxides are effective.

COPPER

Copper is essential, and also has an RDA of only 2 mg. There is only a mere 150 mg in the human body. As a heavy metal, this can be toxic at only 15 mg a day, but that intake is very unlikely. Americans, probably, only take in about half of what they need. Studies have shown low copper is common in those with high blood lipids. Whole grains and beans are the best source. The refined foods we eat cause common deficiencies. There is an important zinc-to-copper ratio. The known biological needs for copper are far too numerous to list.

Dosage: Taking a 2 mg supplement is good insurance. Citrates, oxides, and gluconates are all very absorbable forms to use.

SILICON

Silcon is the ignored, or "orphan element", and almost never found in mineral supplements. More proof that megacorporations have no research departments, only advertising budgets. There is no RDA set for this. Do not use horsetail as a source. Silica levels in our foods vary so greatly, that it is very difficult to say which foods are good sources. Bone and joint health depend on silica as a basic building block. The science here is most impressive. It is very hard to find a supplement with silicon. This is one of the two non-metallic elements we need.

Dosage: Take 10 mg a day, a safe and effective dose. Plain silica gel (silicic acid) is a good, effective, inexpensive source.

IODINE

Iodine is very important, and the only other non-metallic element we need to supplement. It is essential. Eating sea vegetables regularly, like kelp, hijike, and nori, as many Asians do, is not a good idea, surprisingly. All seaweeds contain extreme amounts of iodine. Overdoses of any mineral will unbalance your metabolism, and are not merely excreted without effect. The most important value here is thyroid metabolism. There are only about 30 mg in our bodies, and three-fourths of it is in our thyroid gland. Only 30 mg! Iodine supplements will not correct low T3, or T4 levels, or any thyroid problems however. Only real thyroid hormones will do that.

Dosage: The RDA is a mere 150mcg (micrograms).

CHROMIUM

Chromium is essential. This is often deficient in our diet, due to refining the grains we eat. This is critical for normal blood fat levels, as well as proper blood sugar metabolism. One reason for the epidemic of diabetes and insulin resistance is the widespread deficiency of chromium. Some studies estimate that 9 percent of Americans are, in fact, deficient. This is usually found in mineral supplements. Do not listen to advertisements claiming their form of chromium is the "only effective one". Regular chelates (a non-metal ion bound to a metal ion for better absorbability) are the best source.

Dosage: The RDA is120 mcg (micrograms). Never exceed an intake of more than 400 mcg.

VANADIUM

Vanadium was ignored by science until very recently. There is no RDA for it, even though it is accepted as essential. Almost no supplements contain this vital element. Vanadium has been shown to be important for cholesterol metabolism. Deficiency is all too common, due to our intake of refined foods. There is now very good science on the importance of vanadium, especially for blood fats and blood sugar dysmetabolism. Make sure you get at least 1 mg a day.

Dosage: Take 1 mg (1,000 mcg) a day. Do not exceed 2 mg a day, as this is toxic in excess. Chelates and sulfates are your best choices here.

MOLYBDENUM

Molybdenum is essential. Be sure to take a supplement of this to insure adequate intake. Molybdenum is safe and non-toxic, even though it is a heavy metal. The research is concerned more with soil and plants, rather than animals and humans. We need more human research here. Farmers and gardeners commonly use this in their fertilizer and animal feed.

Dosage: It has a RDA of 75 mcg (micrograms), but that may not be enough. All common salts are good sources, and you will find this in all your supplement formulas.

SELENIUM

Selenium finally has been classified as essential. It was almost ignored until very recently. This is very deficient in our soils and heavily refined foods. Whole grains are the very best source. Studies show people with low blood selenium suffer from higher disease rates such as cancer, coronary heart disease, and diabetes.

Dosage: It has an official RDA of 70 mcg (micrograms). Do not exceed a daily intake of more than 200 mcg; this is a heavy metal and will accumulate in your body. Chelates are the most absorbable form of selenium. Be sure to take this with 200 IU of natural, mixed vitamin E, as they are very synergistic and work together well.

GERMANIUM

Germanium is a very important ultra-trace element, and you will almost never find this in mineral supplements. Clinical human blood studies prove this is a vital, needed element, but our soils and our food are deficient, and it is not found in supplements. Germanium sesquoxide and chelates are safe, but germanium dioxide is not.

Dosage: You only need about 100 mcg of ultra-trace elements like germanium. Do not exceed this amount, as 100 mcg (micrograms) is sufficient.

STRONTIUM

Srontium is another very important trace element, with very good science behind it. You will almost never find this either in mineral supplements Bone and joint health depend on strontium as a building block, as does, calcium absorption. No RDA has been set, but science finally recognizes this as essential.

Dosage: Taking 1 mg (1,000 mcg) is a good dose. Chelates and asparates are good choices. Look for a mineral supplement that has 1 mg of strontium. Do not confuse this with the radioactive form strontium-90.

NICKEL

Nickel is an ignored ultra-trace element. Food and blood analysis of animals and humans show this is an essential element. However, there is little research on the benefits, or for the problems caused by deficiency. The research is mostly for soil and crops. Nickel is essential in human and animal nutrition. You will rarely see this in the mineral supplements on the market.

Dosage: Take 100 mcg (micrograms). Regular salts such as chlorides and sulfates are good.

TIN

Tin is also ignored as a necessary ultra-trace element. Common food and soil studies prove this is an essential element. Most of the research has been concerned with tin toxicity from industrial pollution, instead of the benefits. The FDA irrationally limits the dose to 30 mcg. You almost never find this in mineral supplements. Human studies have shown low blood tin levels in some illnesses, but more research is needed.

Dosage: Take 100 mcg. Regular salts such as chlorides and sulfates are well absorbed.

COBALT

Cobalt is almost never found in mineral supplements, even though it is the basic building block for vitamin B-12. Food and blood studies prove its importance. We are supposed to synthesize our own B-12, but cannot without cobalt in our blood. We probably only take in about 25 mcg or less, but that is enough. This may not sound like much, but we only need to make about 3 mcg of B-12 daily. It must be emphasized that sufficient B-12 is just not found in foods, it is orally unavailable, and a cobalt supplement is the best way to insure the synthesis of the 3 mcg you need every day. There is good science behind cobalt, even in this tiny 25 mcg amount.

Dosage: Taking B-12 orally just doesn't work, so you should take 1 mg of methyl cobalamin.

CESIUM

Cesium is an important ultra-trace mineral. Human blood, common food, and soil studies prove how vital this is for our health. You will almost never find this in mineral supplements. International studies show the importance of cesium in our soil, our food, and our blood. Cesium is essential for humans and animals. Soon science will admit this, and set an RDA. Regular salts, especially chloride, work well here.

Dosage: Taking 100 mcg (micrograms) is all you need. Do not take more than this.

RUBIDIUM

Robidium is not an ultra-trace element at all. Science needs to recognize this is a vital *trace* (not ultra-trace) element. Rubidium deficiency has not been demonstrated. *This is very ignored by science.* Found abundantly in soil, crops, as well in mammals and humans. This is definitely required in human, animal, and plant nutrition. Rubidium is found in fruits, vegetables, poultry, and seafood.

Dosage: Our intake is about 1 mg (1,000 mcg). Rubidium chloride is a good form to use.

GALLIUM

Gallium is an important ultra-trace element. Soil, plant, animal, and human blood studies all show this is vital to our health. The best information was in the book *Advances in Micronutrient Research.* A Japanese study showed people were taking in a mere 12 micrograms of gallium a day. This is an overlooked element for human nutrition.

Dosage: A good dose is 100 mcg (micrograms).

OTHER ELEMENTS

Barium has a lot of research in plant and animal metabolism, thus providing evidence as being essential, especially since we take in about 1,000 mcg a day. This is not an ultra-trace element as it is commonly considered. *Europium* has been shown to extend lifespan in test animals, and more research will be forthcoming. *Indium* is claimed to be beneficial on Internet promotions, but so far there is nothing to validate it. *Lanthanum,* surprisingly, has considerable research and, soon, may well be shown to be essential.

Lanthanum has been shown to increase crop yields, along with other rare earth elements. *Lithium* is definitely essential, but there doesn't seem to be a deficiency of it in our diets. The "therapy" of giving people with bipolar disorders 1,000 times the needed amount is patently insane. *Titanium* has a surprising amount of research available, and will soon be recognized as a necessary element. *Praseodymium* has studies indicating benefits in animals and humans, and one study found 7 pg/ml in human blood. *Samarium* also shows potential as a nutrient in plant and crop studies. One analysis found 3 pg/ml in human blood. *Thulium* (not to be confused with thallium) has a scarcity of research, yet a few soil and plant studies indicate it may be a necessary element. *Yttrium* may also turn out to be essential, although there just isn't enough known about it so far. *Cerium* was found in very large amounts in human blood (170 pg/ml) in a Japanese study. This is a very large amount and probably very meaningful. *Neodymium* was found in very significant amounts, (20 pg/ml), in the same study, and has potential in both animal and human health. Similarly, *Erbium* was found to be 5 pg/ml, indicating this may also be essential. *Dysprosium* was found in 5 pg/ml amounts, and has promise as well. *Tungsten* may well be another necessary ultra-trace element.

CONCLUSION

It may be challenging to find the right supplements for you, but your health is worth it, and now you know how to choose the safest and most effective mineral supplements. Just remember that we need ALL the known and proven elements, and not just the most well-known of them. All minerals work together harmoniously as a team together in concert. Still, it is always worth remembering how dangerous it can be to take supplements when you don't really understand the ingredients. So always read the label! Find a comprehensive mineral formula and take it daily. Remember we are all mineral deficient. All diseases and medical conditions are due in part to mineral deficiency.

8. Beta-Sitosterol

What is beta-sitosterol? It's a phytosterol, or plant alcohol, that is literally in every vegetable in our diet. We already eat this every day, but *just don't get enough of it*. The typical American is estimated to eat only 200 to 400 mg a day, while vegetarians probably eat twice as much. This is surely one of the many reasons vegetarians are healthier and live longer. In fact, studies at the University of Oulu in Finland and the University of Tubingen in Germany prove exactly that. People with high blood sterol levels enjoy better health and longer life. Actually, the term "beta-sitosterol," in commerce, refers to the natural combination of beta-sitosterol, stigmasterol, campesterol, and brassicasterol. This is how they are found naturally in plants. There are no magic foods with high levels of phytosterols, but these can be inexpensively extracted from sugar cane pulp, pine oil, or soybeans.

BETA-SITOSTEROL CAN LOWER YOUR CHOLESTEROL

If there was only one supplement you should take to normalize your cholesterol, it should be beta-sitosterol. Beta-sitosterol is the safest, most studied, proven, and effective single way known to lower total and LDL cholesterol. Even the FDA has approved claims for the prevention of heart disease in general. The studies on this in the medical journals actually go back fifty years, yet most people have never even heard of it. *The published human clinical research is just overwhelming here!* Every year even more studies are published showing the value of plant sterols. Our only good source is green and yellow vegetables, and we just don't eat enough green and yellow vegetables. Taking 300 to 600 mg doses of mixed sterols every day will do wonders for you. If you have a more serious problem you can take three capsules a day, or 900 mg, but only for a year.

BETA-SITOSTEROL CAN REDUCE THE RISK OF HEART AND ARTERY DISEASE

The scientific community has been well aware of plant sterols, and has done extensive studies on humans. This includes gall bladder, bile, and liver functions, since these are all part of the cholesterol metabolism. The major theory of effectiveness is in simply preventing dietary cholesterol from being absorbed in the intestines, where fat is digested. Another way it works is by increasing the flow of bile acids. These acids bind cholesterol in the digestive tract, and excrete it in the feces. There are just too many studies to count, so we'll concentrate on the reviews and the best of the studies. The international research really is overwhelming.

Reviews are always much more informative than single studies. Doctors at the University School of Medicine in Missouri (*Current Atherosclerosis Reports* v 86, 2006) did a similar review. They found the same basic results. At the Third Military Medical University in China a review was done of some of the many studies done in America and Europe (*Chongqing Yixue* v 35, 2006). They found plant sterols to be the most effective, least expensive, and safest way to lower cholesterol levels. The famous Oxford University (*Atherosclerosis Supplements* v 3, 2002) reviewed some of the many published studies. They concluded, "Used as a functional food, sterols could potentially reduce the risk of cardiovascular disease by up to 25 percent." Just imagine reducing heart and artery disease by a full 25 percent by taking a natural, safe, proven, and inexpensive plant ingredient.

A long 16 page review was published in *Nutrition Research* (v 25, 2005) from the Wistar Institute in Philadelphia. They said (in 2005), "Phytosterols have been used as a blood cholesterol lowering agents for the last half century. They have been shown to be effective and safe." The doctors at Kyushu University in Japan (*Foods and Food Ingredients* v 210, 2005) did another fine review. They said, "Plant sterols are natural hypocholesterolemic compounds that lower blood total and LDL cholesterol levels, and hence atherosclerotic risk." Meta-analysis are "super reviews," and rather rare. One was done at the Hartford Hospital (*Diabetes Research* v 84, 2009). "Upon meta-analysis of plant sterols, we saw significantly reduced total and LDL cholesterol levels." At McGill University, in Montreal, (*Canadian Journal of Physiology* v 75, 1997) doctors did a review of eighteen studies, with forty references. They concluded, "The addition to diet of phytosterols represents an effective means of improving circulating lipid profiles to reduce risk of coronary heart disease."

The University of Helsinki took a big interest in lowering cholesterol with plant sterol therapy, back in 1988. The first study (*Clinical Chimica Acta* v 178) studied familial (genetic) hypercholesteremia. The higher the sterol levels they found in the patient's blood, the more cholesterol was excreted, rather than absorbed. The second study was in 1989 (*Metabolism Clinical & Experimental* v 38). Men were again studied for blood levels of sterols and they found the same phenomenon. The third study in 1994 (*American Journal of Clinical Nutrition* v 59) studied vegetarians, who eat about twice as many plant sterols as normal people. They showed that one reason vegetarians have lower cholesterol levels is the efficiency of their cholesterol excretion, due to their intakes of plant sterols. Genetically high cholesterol was again dramatically lowered in families by simply feeding them mixed sterols (*Journal of Laboratory & Clinical Medicine* v 143, 2004). The last study in 1999 (*Current Opinion Lipidology* v 10) said, "Plant sterols may be useful for the treatment of hypercholesteremia . . .they may have a potent cholesterol lowering effect as shown in normal and hypercholesteremic men and women with and without coronary heart disease and diabetes mellitus."

BETA-SITOSTEROL CAN LOWER BLOOD FATS

The best published review of all was from the University of British Columbia (*American Journal of Medicine* v 107, 1999). This included a full eighty-six references. They reviewed sixteen major human studies since 1951 that used plant sterols to lower cholesterol and triglycerides. "In sixteen recently published human studies that used phytosterols to decrease plasma cholesterol levels, in a total of five-hundred nine subjects, phytosterol therapy was accompanied by an average 10 percent decrease in total cholesterol, and 13 percent decrease in LDL cholesterol." They found this worked best with high-fat diets; the worse the diet, the better the results the researchers got. This is the best review to date. In 2004 the same university (*Nutraceutical Science* v 1) did a sixty-three page review, "Role of Plant Sterols in Cholesterol Lowering." This massive work validated the results of the previous studies.

Again, at McGill University (*Metabolism Clinical & Experimental* v. 47, 1998) patients on a fixed diet were given sterols from pine oil for a mere ten days in a strict, randomized crossover study. These were not low-fat or low-cholesterol diets at all. The patients successfully lowered both their total cholesterol and LDL levels in this short term placebo controlled experiment. The doctors concluded, "These results demonstrate the short-term efficacy of pine oil plant sterols as cholesterol lowering agents." At the famous Brandeis University, doctors gave sterols to men in a crossover study, and lowered total cholesterol 10 percent, and LDL a full 15 percent in only four weeks, with no change at all in diet (*Journal of Nutrition* v 134, 2004). Imagine the results if they had also adopted a low-fat diet. This is amazing, and proves you don't need toxic drugs to lower blood fats.

So called "complimentary medicine" doctors have learned adding phytosterols to their usual prescription statin drugs, makes the drugs far more effective, and the toxic dosages can be lowered. This is NOT the point of this book at all. Complimentary medicine is an oxymoron. You can't go right and left at the same time. Statin drugs are so dangerous that liver function tests must be given periodically, to make sure the liver isn't damaged too much. People with liver problems cannot take these drugs.

At the University of California Davis (*Arteriosclerosis and Metabolic Research* v 24, 2004) healthy subjects were given sterols in orange juice for eight weeks with great success. "Sterol orange juice supplementation significantly decreased total (7.2 percent), LDL (12.4 percent) and non-HDL (7.8 percent) cholesterol compared with baseline and with placebo orange juice." Remember these were healthy people with no elevated blood fats.

CONCLUSION

We could go on all day with published studies like this from well known clinics and hospitals around the world. The research is so extensive and wide-ranging over the last thirty years. How something so studied, proven, effective, and well known to the scientific and medical communities, has stayed outside of public knowledge is hard to believe. You will notice that the expensive, prescription, patented, cholesterol drugs are the primary means used to lower cholesterol. There is just no profit in a natural, unpatentable, non-prescription plant extract. It still is not easy to find good beta-sitosterol supplements with realistic amounts of sterols. You can find inexpensive brands, containing the 300 mg, if you search the Internet under "beta-sitosterol."

Many studies have been done in other areas of illness that found beta-sitosterol has great potential in many conditions such as prostate disease, diabetes, blood clotting, ulcers, cancer prevention, tumors, immunity, inflammation, and other conditions. You will see more research and more benefits for beta-sitosterol every year.

9. Flax Oil and Omega-3 Fatty Acids

The most important elements in achieving and maintaining healthy cholesterol levels are diet and exercise. A healthy diet should consist of a balance of omega-3 and omega-6 fatty acids. It is important to have a proper ratio of omega-3 and omega-6 fatty acids in the diet. It is very basic and important to understand that we eat far too many omega-6 fatty acids, and too few omega-3 fatty acids. Our dietary ratio of omega-6 fatty acids to omega-3 fatty acids is too high. We should have about a four-to-one ratio, but actually we have about a twenty-to-one ratio. We eat few foods that contain the omega-3s. This imbalance increases inflammation. Research shows that omega-3 fatty acids reduce inflammation and may help lower risk of chronic diseases.

SOURCES FOR OMEGA-3 FATTY ACIDS

There have been countless studies published on the benefits of omega-3 supplementation. This includes diseases and conditions of all types, and not just blood lipids. It is very difficult to get a good supply of omega-3 fats in your diet, unless you eat a lot of fatty fish like sardines, salmon, herring and mackerel. Another way is to eat a lot of grass fed beef or lamb. These are obviously not good answers. Nor do you need to take expensive EPA (eicosapentaenoic acid) and DHA (docosahexaenoic acid) supplements. Most of the studies have, in fact, been based on fish liver oils. However, *the best source in the world is flaxseed.* Any study using fish liver oils would have gotten the same results with flax oil. Fish oil has dangerous arachidonic acid, and is more subject to oxidation. Flax is a cleaner, much tastier, less expensive plant product that is preferable to fish, krill, squid, or hemp oils. Flax oil is the only source containing vital lignans. Lignans, per se, have very powerful benefits for our health. Flax oil contains an average of about 57 percent omega-3s, while fish oil only about 25 percent. *Buy refrigerated "high lignan" flax oil, and store it refrigerated,* or it will oxidize. You can also use freshly ground flaxseed in your food, but this is not very practical. The omega-6 fatty acids are known as linoleic (LA), while the omega-3s are known as linolenic (ALA). Flax is the best source of ALA, which converts in the body to both DHA and EPA. Flax is also the best source of lignans in the world.

USING FLAX OIL TO LOWER CHOLESTEROL

Let's look at just a few of the human studies using flaxseed to lower cholesterol and triglyceride levels, as well as to improve other important blood parameters. We'll see more studies using flax oil rather than fish oil. A heavily referenced nine page review from the University of Manitoba (*Canadian Journal of Cardiology* v 26, 2010) suggested the use of flax oil to combat the epidemic of coronary heart disease. More and more enlightened doctors are coming to realize the cure for disease is diet and lifestyle rather than toxic drugs. A ten page most impressive meta-analysis was published in the *American Journal of Clinical Nutrition* (v 90, 2009). Five Chinese clinics cooperated in this endeavor. They suggested flaxseed and flaxseed oil be used to prevent all forms of heart and artery disease as regular therapy.

At the University of Toronto (*American Journal of Clinical Nutrition* v 69, 1999) flaxseed without oil (defatted) in muffins lowered both total and LDL cholesterol levels in both men and women. If they had used whole flax with oil, the results would have been even more dramatic. The Indian diet is far superior to the American diet overall, as it is based on grains and vegetables basically. At the National Institute of Nutrition in India (*Nutrition Research* v 12, 1992) people were given high omega-3 canola and mustard seed oil in their diets. Their TC and TG levels dropped, while other blood qualities were improved. They suggested that canola and mustard oils be used in the daily diet to supply the ALA. At PSG College in India (*Indian Journal of Nutrition* v 42, 2005), elderly people with high cholesterol were given flax oil. This lowered their total cholesterol, LDL and triglycerides, and raised their HDL. The doctors concluded, "Flax oil supplementation has a beneficial effect on the lipoid profile of the elderly." At Nikea Hospital in Greece (*Atherosclerosis* v 167, 2003) dyslipidemic people lowered their CRP levels a whopping 38 per cent on average with flax oil. This is amazing. CRP, homocysteine, and uric acid are the other three CHD diagnostic markers besides total cholesterol and triglycerides. They also lowered other vital inflammatory markers. "Linseed oil lowered inflammatory markers in these patients." The CHD death rate in all countries could be lowered significantly, if everyone simply took flax oil daily.

A fine book, *Flaxseed in Human Nutrition* (AOCS Press) was published in 2003. In there is a fourteen page review of atherosclerosis. They claim taking a whole flax supplement daily will reduce the development of atherosclerosis by an amazing 69 percent. "Whole flax reduces the development of atherosclerosis by 69 percent, and this reduction is associated with a reduction in serum total cholesterol, and LDL. Why are we using expensive, toxic, harmful drugs when we have an inexpensive natural remedy that does so much better?

At Roman City Hospital (*Revisto Medico* v 109, 2005) forty hyperlipidemic patients were given flax supplements for sixty days. The doctors summarized, "Dietary flaxseed significantly improves lipid profile in hyperlipidemic patients, and may favorably modify cardiovascular risk factors." At St. Boniface Hospital a wonderful review (*Applied Physiology and Nutrition Metabolism* v 34, 2009) was done of twenty-eight human flaxseed studies. They clearly found, "Flaxseed significantly reduced circulating total and LDL concentrations."

At the University of Regensburg (*American Journal of Cardiology* v 76, 1995), in Germany, thirty-five men with heart disease, in a double blind study, were given vegetable based canola or fish oil based omega-3s. Both groups lowered their total cholesterol, LDL and triglyceride levels. This is an excellent study that demonstrates whichever the source, fish or plant, the benefits still occur equally. *Flax is the best source of all.*

A study at the University of North Dakota (*American Journal of Clinical Nutrition* v 88 2008) proved that both fish and flax oil are both good sources of omega-3s. Men were divided into six groups and given fish, flax, or sunflower oil (placebo). Blood levels of both EPA and DHA were increased in the men taking fish or flax oils. "ALA is the direct precursor of both EPA and DHA." Another study at the University of Surrey (*Atherosclerosis* v 181, 2005) got the same results. Patients were given fish, flax, and sunflower oils in a placebo controlled study. Blood levels of EPA and DHA increased significantly. Their levels of total cholesterol fell 12.3 percent with flax oil, but only 7.6 percent with fish oil. Triglycerides fell, an amazing, 23 percent overall!

Postmenopausal women, at the University of Oklahoma, were given ground flaxseed for three months in a double blind study (*Journal of Clinical Endocrinology* v 87, 2002). They lowered both their total and LDL cholesterol by 6.0 percent, with no change in diet or exercise. They lowered their triglycerides a whopping 12.8 percent with no other treatments. This is most impressive! Flax oil really is amazing. This is a supplement for everyone, including you children and pets. *You must buy refrigerated "high lignan" flax oil and keep it refrigerated.* Take one to two capsules, or one-half teaspoon of liquid (1.5 g).

OTHER BENEFITS OF OMEGA-3 FATTY ACIDS

It is very difficult to reduce blood pressure in people simply by using natural supplements. Generally, the only way to lower blood pressure is a total program of diet and lifestyle with regular exercise. About one-fourth of Americans have high blood pressure. More and more younger people suffer from this every year. At the University of Trondheim, in Norway, doctors gave omega-3 fatty acid supplements to men with high blood pressure. There were no other treatments, or changes in their lifestyles (*Proceedings of the Scandinavian Symposium on Lipids 16th,* 1991). Amazingly enough, they lowered their blood pressure just from taking the omega-3 supplements! This kind of study is most significant. Hypertension causes strokes and early death, and is correlated with insulin resistance. Hypertension is an epidemic in most of the world.

At the Women's University (*Nippon Eiyo* v 49, 1996), in Japan, fifty healthy young women, with no heart or circulatory problems, were studied for a wide variety of diets ranging from 15 to 40 percent fat calories. Their diets literally and directly determined the quality of their blood, especially the ratio of omega-3 fatty acids to omega-6 fatty acids. The women with the highest levels of omega-3s, and the lowest levels of omega-6s, had the lowest TC and TG levels, and the highest HDL levels. This study shows the effect of diet on blood parameters using direct laboratory measurements in normal people.

At the University of Pennsylvania (*Nutrition Reviews* v 62, 2004) a very nice review was done for nine different flax oil studies. The authors found up to an 18 percent reduction in both total and LDL cholesterol from simple flax supplementation in humans. They also found other benefits such as lowering blood sugar. Again, at this university (*Journal of the American College of Nutrition* v 27, 2008) men given flax supplements improved their cholesterol profile along with other CHD benefits, such as improving insulin sensitivity. In this same journal (v 12, 1993), at the Jordan Heart Fund, flaxseed was given to people in whole wheat bread. "Total and LDL cholesterol fell significantly." Other parameters improved as well, such as reduction of lipid oxidation.

CONCLUSION

Omega-3 fatty acids are considered to be necessary fatty acids. They have shown positive effects in helping to lower your cholesterol and with other health issues. Mounting evidence has proven that inflammation plays an important part in many chronic diseases such as heart disease, arthritis, asthma, diabetes, and most cancers. The omega-3 fatty acids have proven to be essential in reducing inflammation. They are needed to maintain a healthy body, but the body can't produce them, we need to supply our bodies with this important nutrient. Studies have proven that flaxseed oil is by far the best source of omega-3 fatty acids, and omega-3 fatty acids have proven to be instrumental in lowering your cholesterol.

10. Beta Glucan

A strong immune system is vital to the preservation of your good health. Beta gulcan is a naturally derived polysaccharide which has been studied for its immune stimulating properties, and the properties to improve the levels of your total cholesterol. Due to the gel-like substance that is produced from beta glucan when it is dissolved in the digestive tract, it can be effective in reducing the overall cholesterol in the body. A substantial body of evidence indicates that beta glucan, or foods containing it can be effective in your overall health.

BETA GLUCAN AS AN IMMUNE SYSTEM STIMULANT AND ENHANCER

Beta glucan is the most powerful immune system stimulant known to science including any pharmaceutical drugs, like interferon-alpha. It is a polysaccharide found in oats, barley, yeast, and mushrooms. The miraculous powers of beta glucan to lower cholesterol and triglycerides, and strengthen our immune systems, have been known about for more than three decades. At the University of Hamburg, in Germany, it was shown that *all 1,3 configuration beta glucans have the same biological potency whether they are derived from oats or yeast*, which are the two major sources (*Carbo-*

Lower Your Cholesterol Without Drugs

hydrate Research v 297, 1997). *Basically, they are all true 1,3 beta glu-cans.* Do not listen to advertisements that tell you one is better than the other, in order to sell their product. You need at least 200 mg a day of actual glucan to be effective. You can now get sixty capsules for only ten dollars. You can take twice this much for a year, if you are treating a health condition. It has only been since the year 2000 that technology finally provided inexpensive, strong beta glucan to consumers. Eat oatmeal three times a week, and you won't need to take beta glucan supplements.

Beta glucan is the most powerful immunity enhancer known to science, regardless of cost. There are many studies, on animals and humans that show the great value it has to strengthen our immune systems, and even the potential to help against tumors and cancer growth. At the University of Saskatchewan, in Cana-da, (*Microbiology & Immunity* v 41, 1997) researchers showed its power to stimulate the immune system. Other studies have found such potential uses as fighting infections, improving intestinal flora, irritable bowel syndrome, diabetic conditions, healing ulcers, and better digestion. There are many, many stud-ies on blood lipids, so we'll just talk about some of the more interesting human published ones.

Beta glucan strengthens our immune system. This gives us optimum healing power in our body to fight off infections of all kinds. You should understand that it is very difficult to study human beings for immune function. Animal studies are used, because you just can't infect humans with deadly micro-organisms, give half of them beta glucan, and see who lives and who doesn't. Animal studies have shown results for such conditions as various cancers, infections, tumors, diabetes, digestion, intestinal function, and ulcers. Finally, since 2000, we are seeing many human studies published, where real people can safely be used.

At the University of Saskatchewan, beta glucan protected mice from deadly injections of Staphalococcus aureus. In another study there, mice were injected with equally deadly

76

Eimeria vermiformis, but beta glucan protected them. In a third study, mice were given the toxic drug dexamethasone, and then injected with the deadly Eimeria virus. Even after their immune systems were impaired by the drug, the beta glucan protected them. At SRI International, the Euglena gracilis virus was injected into various test animals, but beta glucan stopped them from dying. At the University of Kansas, pigs were given deadly Staphalococcus suis, but beta glucan saved them. The doctors there did an in-depth study of various immune system markers to discover the mechanisms by which it worked.

BETA GLUCAN CAN LOWER YOUR CHOLESTEROL

At Harvard Medical School, in Massachusetts (*Critical Reviews in Food Science & Nutrition* v 39, 1999), doctors found that both oat and yeast beta glucans lowered serum cholesterol levels, with no change in diet. In their words, "In addition to decreasing the intake of total fat, saturated fat, and dietary cholesterol, blood serum, cholesterol can be further decreased by dietary fiber, especially from sources rich in beta glucan such as oats and yeast."

At the University of Syracuse, in New York seventy-one men and women, with high cholesterol, were given various combinations of low-fat diets or regular diets, with and without oat beta glucan. In four weeks, total cholesterol levels were reduced as much as 17 percent, and HDL levels increased (*Journal of the American Dietary Association* v 90, 1990).This shows the benefit of making better food choices, along with taking proven supplements.

At the University of Massachusetts (*American Journal of Clinical Nutrition* v 70, 1999), researchers found that giving yeast beta glucan to obese men, with high cholesterol, lowered both their total and LDL levels by a full 8 percent, with no change in diet. They summarized the study: "Thus, the yeast derived beta glucan fiber lowered the total cholesterol concentrations, and was well-tolerated." As usual, the "side effects" were all positive in nature.

At the U. S. Human Nutrition Research Center in Maryland, (*Journal of Nutritional Biochemistry* v 8, 1997), people were given oat beta glucan. This lowered their cholesterol levels, with no changes in diet or exercise. They also found that other metabolic conditions improved; new benefits of beta glucan are always being discovered. Again, at the Human Nutrition Research Center (*Journal of the American College of Nutrition* v 16, 1997), men and women, with high blood lipid levels, were given oat beta glucan in a crossover study. After only five weeks, the groups were switched, and those getting the beta glucan just received only the usual American diet. Both total cholesterol and LDL levels decreased significantly. In their words, "A significant dose response, due to beta glucan concentration in the oat extract, was observed in the total cholesterol levels." A third study was done there (*American Journal of Clinical Nutrition* v 80, 2004), with barley beta glucan. This lowered the subjects LDL and total cholesterol. Thorough studies like these, with real people at the most prestigious research centers in the world, leave no doubt about the power of beta glucan to lower blood fats.

At Industrial Research Limited in New Zealand (*Carbohydrate Polymers* v 29, 1996) researchers used barley derived beta glucan to try and understand the actual metabolic mechanisms by which it lowered blood fats. They discovered that it increased the secretion of bile acids from the gall bladder. At the Netherlands Maastricht University (*American Journal of Clinical Nutrition* v 78, 2003), people were given oat beta glucan. This lowered their cholesterol in only three weeks. Another study there, in the same journal (v 83, 2006), got identical results. Again, at Maastricht (*Journal of Nutrition* v 137, 2007) oat beta glucan lowered total cholesterol and LDL levels in four weeks. Hypercholesterolemic children, at Radiant Research, were given beta glucan to get dramatic improvements in only four weeks (*Nutrition Research* v 23, 2003). At the University of Minnesota (*Nutrition Journal* v 6, 2007), men and women were given oat beta glucan for three weeks. Total and LDL cholesterol were significantly reduced. Two studies were published in *JAMA* (v 265, 1991 and v 267, 1992), where adults were given oat beta glucan and lowered their cholesterol in weeks. This was with no change in diet or exercise.

At the University of Lund, in Sweden, (*Annals of Nutrition & Metabolism* v 43, 1999), sixty-six mildly hypercholesterolemic men were given oat milk, high in beta glucan, every day for five weeks. This was a classic double blind study, where half the men received rice milk with no beta glucan. Of course, the men getting the oat milk lowered their total cholesterol. The doctors said, "It is concluded that oat milk has cholesterol reducing properties." They did another study (*European Journal of Clinical Nutrition* v 59, 2005), and gave oat glucan to patients. This improved their cholesterol, as well as their glucose metabolism, in just eight weeks.

You can see from studies like these, there is no doubt that beta glucan is a safe, effective, powerful, proven, and inexpensive way to lower your cholesterol levels. Yet, most people have never even heard of it. Many vitamin companies don't even sell it. It can be difficult to find a reliable, strong, inexpensive brand with 200 mg or more, even in the health food stores. However, you can search the internet to look for a reliable brand. Many people insist on taking dangerous, expensive, prescription drugs, when they can use natural remedies like beta glucan. The use of statin drugs now is epidemic. This is an unnecessary epidemic.

BETA GLUCAN CAN PREVENT AND TREAT CANCER

At the Mayo Clinic, lung cancer in mice was reduced by beta glucan. At Tokyo College, doctors found strong antitumor properties for beta glucan. At Tokyo University, doctors found anticancer activity in mice, when given beta glucan. They suggested it be used as a biological response modifier in human cancer patients. At Wuhan University, doctors found powerful antitumor activity in mice given beta glucan. At the University of Louisville, they found the antitumor effect of beta glucan was largely due to enhancing beneficial natural killer (NK) cells. This is a proven basic supplement for children and adults. Even your pets should be taking this daily for the same reasons.

CONCLUSION

There are numerous beta glucan benefits. As cited in this chapter, studies have shown that taking beta glucan can potentially reduce a person's chances of developing an infectious illness, or other conditions that compromise the functioning of the immune system. Beta glucan is prescribed to patients by many health care professionals to prevent, and to fight cancer. One of the most noted benefits of beta glucan is to help lower bad cholesterol. Oat derived beta glucan significantly improves HDL cholesterol and diminishes LDL cholesterol.

11. Soy Isoflavones

Soy isoflavones have finally seen a lot of research regarding their health benefits. These impressive studies demonstrate the cholesterol lowering benefits of soy isoflavones. Eating more soy foods is a fine thing to do, but it may not be easy for most Westerners. Tofu is a very highly refined food. Soy yogurt contains sugar. Soy sauce is a mere condiment. Tempeh, annato, seitan, soy flour, soy sprouts, boiled soybeans, and soy cheese are just not popular foods outside of Asia. However, if you use soymilk you are getting enough isoflavones. Using soy milk and taking isoflavone supplements are a much more practical and realistic means of isoflavone intake. A supplement with 40 mg of genestein and daidzein is a good addition to get what you need.

WHAT ARE ISOFLAVONES?

The two main isoflavones we are concerned about here are genestein and daidzein. These are not "phytoestrogens," as you have been told endlessly. There is no such thing as plant hormones. In fact *there is no such thing as a "phytoestrogen."* All hormones come from animals, not plants. There are no plant based hormones, or plant based estrogens, or estrogen mimics. Genestein and daidzein are, in fact, *flavones* and completely unrelated to estrogen or any other hormone. Flavones are plant pigment flavonoids, while estrogens are steroids secreted by the endocrine (ductless) glands in animals. The research on soy and blood fats is simply overwhelming. There are just countless studies on the benefits of isoflavones for most every medical condition. New ones appear in the journals every week. We are therefore going to concentrate on the meta-analysis and reviews.

SOY ISOFLAVONES CAN LOWER YOUR CHOLESTEROL

At the Chinese University of Hong Kong (*American Journal of Clinical Nutrition* v 81, 2005) a meta-analysis was done for twenty-three different published clinical trials. "Soy protein with intact isoflavones was associated with significant decreases in total cholesterol (3.77 percent), LDL cholesterol (5.255 percent), and triglycerides (7.27 percent) and increases in HDL cholesterol (3.03 percent). This is simply amazing, the study showed positive results with just soy supplementation. Why are doctors giving people toxic, expensive prescription drugs, when we have safe, inexpensive, natural, proven natural supplements? The answer in one word is "money."

The well known Anderson Meta-Analysis was done at the Veterans Medical Center in Kentucky (*New England Journal of Medicine* v 333, 1995). Dr. Anderson and his associates reviewed a stunning thirty-eight published trials. "In this meta-analysis we found the consumption of soy protein, rather than animal protein, significantly decreased serum concentrations of total cholesterol, LDL cholesterol, and triglycerides."

At the National Institute of Health and Nutrition in Tokyo (*American Journal of Clinical Nutrition* v 85, 2007), a meta-analysis was done of eleven randomized controlled studies. "Soy isoflavones significantly decreased serum total, and LDL cholesterol." They compared plain isoflavones, soy protein with isoflavones, and soy protein enriched with isoflavones. The enriched protein decreased LDL cholesterol by a full 5 percent, and increased the HDL cholesterol by a full 3 percent. Whole enriched soy was the most effective form to use. At the Medical Centre of Hong Kong (*Nutrition Journal* v 2, 2003), another meta-analysis of seventeen published clinical trials were carefully reviewed and chosen. Again, they found the whole soy foods, whole soy protein, and enriched soy protein to be the most effective in lowering blood fats.

OTHER BENEFITS OF SOY ISOFLAVONES

A fine ten page review was done at the University of Toronto (*Phytoestrogens and Health* 2002). They found the worldwide literature clearly supports the value of soy foods to lower cardiovascular risks in general. They also found great value in treating other various diseases such as osteroporosis and cancer. Another review came from the University of Milano. Here (*British Journal of Nutrition* 97, 2007), they were most impressed by the Anderson Meta-Analysis of 1995 listed above. These doctors actually found thirty-three new studies after 1995. They compared these to the thirty-eight trials Anderson did, and concluded, "The re-evaluation thus shows that the thirty-three studies published in the last ten years are in agreement with the Anderson meta-analysis and confirm its validity." So, you have a full seventy-one international studies confirming the value of soy. These doctors deserve a lot of credit for such excellent work.

At Harbin Medical University in China (*Jibing Kongzhi Zazhi* v 9, 2005), the doctors reviewed some of the massive literature on the benefits of soy foods for cardiovascular health and lowering cholesterol. They were most impressed by these findings. At White Wave Foods (*Future Lipidology* v 2, 2007), a fine and thorough twenty-page review was done. They mentioned the FDA actually approved a health claim for overall heart and artery health from eating more soyfoods. The FDA actually allows the statement, "The combined cardioprotective attributes of soyfoods warrant their having a larger role in Western diets." At the University of Helsinki (*BioFactors* 22, 2004), a fine review was done. They reviewed studies on the benefits of soy for cardiovascular health, as well as breast and prostate cancer, and found the same results.

We could go on with study after study on real people given soy isoflavone supplements in clinics around the world, but you see these benefits are established clearly in the medical field. Soy isoflavones improve our blood profiles significantly, improve the quality of our arteries, and are even shown to lower blood pressure. All of these effects can be obtained without any change in diet or exercise. When combined with other proven supplements, a low-fat diet, and reasonable exercise (such as walking), the effects are even more dramatic.

CONCLUSION

It has become popular in certain circles, on the Internet, and from some misguided, self-appointed experts to talk about the supposed "dangers" of eating soy foods. This misinformation has become somewhat popular, despite the fact there are never any valid references to verify their claims of "dangerous side effects." The very idea that soy foods have negative effects on our health is simply ludicrous and totally contradicted by science. Any allergies to soy foods are almost non-existent. *All of this propaganda comes from the meat and dairy industries.* It should be obvious that the billions of Asian people, who have eaten soy foods as a basic part of their diets for centuries, never suffer these illusory "side effects." People in Japan, Thailand, China, Viet Nam, Taiwan, and Singapore use soy foods (fermented and unfermented) as staples. Overall they suffer from much less cancer, heart disease, diabetes, obesity, thyroid, and other conditions than Westerners do. The people in Japan are the longest lived and healthiest of all, especially in the rural areas. The Okinawans, specifically, are the healthiest and longest lived people on earth, and eat the most soy foods. The Taiwanese eat huge amounts of soy foods. You can see from the many clinical studies that there are never negative side effects from the patients taking these supplements.

Entire books have been written about the benefits of soy isoflavones for many other conditions. In fact, new studies with more benefits are constantly being published. People are becoming aware that *the real dangers lie in milk and milk products.* All adults of all races are lactose (milk sugar) intolerant. Milk and dairy consumption is down more every year. This is especially true among African and Asian people, who are the most lactose intolerant. Now grocery stores carry more and more soy milk, soy cheese, soy yogurt, soy cream cheese, soy "meats," various forms of tofu, and other soy products all the time. The dairy interests are understandably upset about so many people switching from dairy products to soy products. They are the ones promoting the misinformation campaign about soy foods. This anti-soy propaganda is not from ethical, unbiased scientists; it is from the meat and dairy industries. You will not find any published independent clinical studies showing any negative side effects from soy food consumption.

12. Life Style

Aside from the food we eat every day, let's take a quick look at lifestyle. Bad habits such as smoking, drinking alcohol, drinking coffee, and using recreational drugs obviously worsen your health. Living a stressful life, being overweight, taking prescription drugs, and lack of exercise are additional factors. Let's examine these factors to clearly understand the impact they have on our well-being.

BENEFITS OF EXERCISE

Exercise is the most important life style factor to look at. Do you do physical work at your job? Do you enjoy any sport, like golf or tennis that gives you a workout every week? Do you belong to a gym, or have workout equipment in your home? Are you a member of an indoor swimming pool? Do you take a walk every day? *Walking* is the most practical, most effective, and most enjoyable exercise for many people. You can lower your blood lipids, as well as lower your blood pressure, with no change in diet simply by walking a half hour a day. Studies abound on the cholesterol lowering benefits of any exercise, even for young people.

At the University Medical School, in Turkey, (*Indian Journal of Physiology & Pharmacology* v 43, 1999) it was shown that men, of any age, who exercised regularly had lower total cholesterol, lower LDL levels, higher HDL levels, less body fat, and all over less risk for coronary heart disease. At the University of Maryland (*Medical Science Sports Exercise* v 26, 1994), a ten month, long-term study was done on older obese men. They used a combination of low-calorie diet and aerobic exercise. Of course the men lost weight and body fat, lowered total, LDL and triglyceride levels, and raised HDL levels. The same university did another long-term, nine month study (*Metabolism & Clinical Experiments* v 48, 1999) on middle-aged, overweight men. This time they put them on the American Heart Association (AHA) diet (which really isn't very strict or hard to follow at all), and had them do aerobic exercise regularly. They got the same results as in the previous study, and the men showed much improved health.

At the Center for Adult Diseases in Osaka (*Domyaku Koka* v 21, 1994), doctors took four hundred and fifty-nine middle aged, healthy men and just had them walk every day. No change in diet, lifestyle, or supplements, just walking. They found their HDL levels went up, and the risk for coronary heart disease went down almost immediately. At the University of Padua, in Italy, (*Journal of Sports Medicine* v 31, 1991) healthy young male and female athletes were given either aerobic or resistance exercise. Clear benefits resulted *no matter what kind of exercise they did*. The usual results of lower TC, LDL, and TG levels, and higher HDL levels were obtained in healthy, young, well-trained athletes. A similar study was done at the University of Vermont (*Metabolism & Clinical Experiment* v. 41, 1992). The researchers again found whether you do aerobic or resistance exercise it just doesn't matter, as you get the same basic cardiovascular benefits. They said, "Aerobically trained and resistance trained young males have comparable, and favorable cardiovascular disease risk profiles compared with untrained males, and this appears to be related to their low level of adiposity (fat mass), and low intake of dietary fat."

At the University of Pittsburgh (*Journal of Sports Medicine* v 35, 1995), groups of both premenopausal and postmenopausal women were asked to walk every day. The postmenopausal women had an average age of fifty-five, and a whopping 38 percent body fat! The doctors said, "A single bout of walking has the potential to acutely affect the blood lipid profile of premenopausal as well as postmenopausal women." At Texas A&M University (*Journal of Applied Physiology* v 79, 1995), middle-aged men were given short-term exercise programs, with the usual beneficial results. The researchers said, "These data show that a single session of exercise, performed by untrained hypercholesterolemic men, alters blood lipid and apolipoprotein concentrations." Please note, they said just one single session. Exercise is powerful therapy.

You already knew that exercise is good for you, and lowers your blood lipids without changing your diet. Think what daily walking will do when you make some changes in your diet and take proven supplements!

TAKING PRESCRIPTION AND RECREATIONAL DRUGS

Americans will down more toxic prescription drugs by far than any other country. The damage from these drugs is incalculable. Over two hundred thousand people die every year from these synthetic abominations. The biggest epidemic now is antidepressant, and other psych medications. Do not take prescription drugs except for rare cases like opiates for temporary pain relief, and insulin for type 1 diabetics with no pancreas. You cannot poison your way to health. There is a natural cure for all your medical conditions.

Americans also use more recreational drugs by far than any other country. Marijuana is the most used, but has few physical effects fortunately. The negative effects are psychological. Prescription opiates are an epidemic, especially *hydro-codone, the most prescribed drug in America*. This list includes prescription depressants and prescription stimulants. Cocaine is still extremely popular despite its high price. Amphetamines of all types are widely consumed. Ecstasy is very popular. The psychedelic drugs are out of favor for the most part. We are the most drugged up nation on earth. This is simply a symptom of a deep unhappiness and lack of fulfillment in our lives.

SMOKING

One-third American adults smoke. Smoking is correlated with many major diseases such as various cancers. We certainly don't have to argue the case that smoking is deadly. The biggest and most important heart studies, like the Seven Countries Study, and the Helsinki Study, have repeatedly proven this. Smoking worsens your blood lipid profile, is a major factor for coronary heart disease, is an important factor in many other diseases, and shortens your lifespan. The National Cholesterol Education Program published a lengthy report (*Archives of Internal Medicine* v 148, 1988) on all aspects of treating hypercholesterolemia. Examining smoking as a factor, they found that men with the lowest cholesterol levels had only 1.6 deaths per one thousand if they didn't smoke, but 6.3 deaths if they did. Men with the highest cholesterol levels had 6.4 deaths per one thousand if they didn't smoke, but a frightening 21.4 deaths if they did. The problem is that nicotine is so addictive; it is very hard to stop. There is no reason to quote a list of studies here to show what is already obvious. Smoking is a major factor in heart disease, alters our steroid levels, has countless negative effects on our health, and causes early death. If you want to live a long, healthy life of good quality, and avoid heart and artery disease, you have to stop smoking. It is very important to note that when you quit smoking, your health recovers very quickly. You soon approach the same level of CHD (Coronary Heart Disease) risk as those who have never smoked. *It is never too late to quit*, and you can quickly reverse most of the damage you've done.

CAFFEINE

The research has shown that coffee, or any form of caffeine (e.g. energy drinks, guarana, yerba mate) is much more harmful than you might think. Unfiltered, French press, and espresso are even worse because of the toxic oils, cafestol and kaweol. *Caffeine is the most popular psychoactive drug in the world.* It is insidiously addictive, and easy to get hooked on. It is legal, cheap, popular, and socially acceptable. Caffeine has very negative effects on our cholesterol and triglyceride levels. It has even worse effects on our blood sugar and insulin. It contributes to hypertension, which is the most prominent medical condition in the world. Studies proving all this were done at such institutions as the Nordic School of Public Health in Sweden, National Institute of Public Health in the Netherlands, and King's College in London. *Just one cup of coffee, or one dose of caffeine daily, is enough to ruin your health and shorten your life.* If you are addicted to caffeine, admit your dependence and get off of it.

ALCOHOL

We come to a much more complex problem with alcohol. Most all countries on earth have a serious problem with alcohol consumption. *No other drug on earth causes, anywhere near, the damage that overall alcohol consumption does.* Every major study has shown that excessive alcohol consumption (i.e. more than two drinks a day or heavy drinking even once a week) is a major risk for coronary heart disease. Women are much more sensitive to alcohol than men. Ironically, some studies have shown that people who have only one or two drinks a day (and never have more than this), supposedly have less heart disease, better cholesterol levels, and live longer than people who don't drink alcohol at all. *Alcohol, even in moderation, is not part of a healthy lifestyle.* If you only drink one or two drinks a day, you may not hurt your blood lipid profile, or get more heart disease, but it will cause other damage. Drinking more than two drinks a day, or drinking heavily even one day a week, will raise your cholesterol, and you'll have a bigger risk of heart and artery disease. You should be aware that even one or two drinks a day has been shown to put your at higher risk for other diseases. Alcohol is a poison, not a "French Paradox."

CONCLUSION

The evidence for the importance of healthy lifestyles is now overwhelming. Smoking, drinking, drugs, bad nutritional habits, and lack of physical activity are life-style health determinants linked to a number of major health problems, such as cancer, cardio-vascular disease, and obesity. We know that lifestyle-related diseases are placing an increasing burden on health systems around the world. Prevention is the best answer to the problem. We can prevent these diseases by making small changes in our behavior such as our diet, or physical exercise. Making these changes can lead to a healthier life. It's just a matter of commitment.

13. Heredity and High Cholesterol

Some of us cannot maintain a healthy cholesterol profile with just diet and moderate exercise. Diet and lifestyle contribute to the cholesterol level, but sometimes high cholesterol is the result of genetics and may remain high despite a good diet and reasonable exercise. One can have a predisposition to high cholesterol. Genetics can play a role here. There are a good number of people with genetically high cholesterol and triglycerides, over the 300 level. Such people are at severe risk for all forms of CHD, cancer, diabetes, and premature death. Obviously, they need to do more to lower their blood fats. Here, better food choices have to be made, supplements added, weekly fasting, no prescription drugs, drop any bad habits, and do more exercise.

DIET

There is no cholesterol in any plant. Cholesterol is only found in animals and animal products. People who eat a pure vegetarian diet (no eggs or dairy) consume no cholesterol at all. Such people generally have levels of about 150 mg/dL or less, and every milligram of this is manufactured by their livers from the plant foods they eat. People with genetically high cholesterol must stop eating all beef, pork, lamb, poultry, eggs, milk, and dairy products. Seafood can be eaten in moderation as a four-ounce daily portion, if you have no allergy. Choose low-fat fish and shellfish over high-fat fish.

Vegetable oils contain no cholesterol, but *should be very restricted as well*. Vegetable oils also are generally high in omega-6 fatty acids, and low in omega-3 fatty acids. This is another reason to use as little as possible. Americans have an imbalance of omega-6 to omega-3 fatty acids. Flax is the best known source of omega-3 fatty acids, and taking 2.5 grams (1/2 teaspoon) of bulk refrigerated flax oil is recommended for tough cases. Please refer to Chapter 9: Flax Oil.

Milk and dairy products should be avoided entirely. That includes the low-fat and no-fat varieties, lactose-free, skim milk, and yogurt. Dairy products are full of lactose and casein. There are a variety of very good tasting soy, rice, almond, and oat products to replace them. Dairy foods are the most allergenic and harmful food group of all.

SUPPLEMENTS

It is very important that people with very high blood fats take all four of the "cornerstone supplements"—beta-sitosterol, flax oil, beta glucan, and soy isoflavones. It would also be a good idea to double the amount of beta-sitosterol to 600 mg, and double the amount of beta glucan to 400 mg for one year. The guggul gum and soy isoflavones should remain at 250 mg (10 percent sterones) and 40 mg respectively. Guggul should be discontinued after one year.

Many of the other supplements discussed should also be included in your program. This would include acidophilus, beta carotene, vitamin E, FOS, garlic, L-glutamine, and lecithin. Curcumin, aloe vera, guggul gum, guar gum, and citrus pectin for six to twelve months only. These supplements are inexpensive, and generally good for your health in many other ways. Take 3 g of TMG (trimethylglycine) daily for one year to rejuvenate, and clear out your liver. Then take 1 g daily, permanently. Good liver function is vital to healthy blood lipid levels.

BALANCING HORMONES

Hormone balancing is no longer an option. As we discuss in Chapters 15 and 16, you must balance your basic hormones. DHEA and testosterone are the first ones to measure, but do not take these unless you are proven to be low. Melatonin should be used by people over forty. That can be tested at 3:00 AM with saliva if you wish. Transdermal progesterone can be used by both men and women, but in different amounts. Pregnenolone should usually be taken by anyone over the age of forty. If estradiol or estrone levels are too high, in men or women, then changes in diet and lifestyle can lower them. Women should test estriol. Thyroid hormones T3 and T4 should be tested. HGH (Human Growth Hormone) can be used by anyone over the age of fifty, but is very expensive, and should be injected daily. This is the only book to talk about the effects of our hormones on our cholesterol and triglyceride levels. Doctors, even endocrinologists, are completely unaware of this, and don't test hormone levels for high blood fats as they should. Cholesterol is the basic precursor for the other sex hormones.

EXERCISE

Regular physical activity is crucial to lowering your cholesterol. Most health organizations recommend, minimally, thirty minutes a day of moderate to vigorous exercise, such as walking, jogging, biking, or gardening to aid in lowering cholesterol. For those battling genetically high cholesterol, you must get more exercise than other people, every day. Ideally this would be both resistance and aerobic. One way that exercise can help lower cholesterol is by helping you to lose or maintain your weight. Being overweight will increase the amount of LDL in your blood. People with severely high blood fat levels need to get down to a normal weight.

WEEKLY FASTING

It has been proven that routine and periodic fasting lowers blood cholesterol levels. Fasting also reduces blood sugar levels, triglycerides, and weight. Weekly fasting is not an option Fasting, one day a week, drinking only water and eating nothing during a 24-hour period is a great help here. The fasting leads to hunger and, in response, the body releases more cholesterol. Just go from dinner to dinner without eating on one chosen day a week.

CONCLUSION

If genetic abnormalities cause your body to produce excess cholesterol or prevent your body from absorbing it, cholesterol can certainly be harder to manage. However, that doesn't mean it is impossible. It means making an even bigger commitment to a healthy lifestyle. Tough cases need more time, attention, and effort to cure.

14. Low Cholesterol

A high blood cholesterol level increases your risk of many diseases. However, are there risks when your blood cholesterol level is too low? The "ketogenic" diet (also known as Paleolithic or Atkins) advocated eating all the meat and fat you wanted. It was popular to say "cholesterol doesn't matter." Some even claimed that cholesterol should not be, "too low." Of course, this is patently ridiculous. A popular life extension magazine states that the optimal range for serum cholesterol is 180 mg/dL to 200 mg/dL. They further said that cholesterol levels below 180 mg/dL cause an "increased risk of mortality." Asinine!

In this book, you have seen references to the largest and most comprehensive studies on heart and artery health in the world. This includes the Framingham Study, the 17 Countries Study, and the MRFIT Study. Hundreds of thousands of real people proved that you get benefits all the way down to a level of about 150 mg/dL total serum cholesterol. *TC 150 mg/dL is the ideal level.*

AGE

As we reach the age of sixty, we often start losing the ability to synthesize cholesterol. You can find elderly, sickly people who eat a high fat diet, get no exercise, and have very unhealthy lifestyles. Yet, they have rather low cholesterol levels. Therefore, *when we reach old age, our cholesterol levels become less accurate in predicting good heart health.* Lab results become less meaningful. For older people, you have to look at their cholesterol results in light of how they live. This makes it even more important to eat a low-fat diet, exercise, take effective supplements, balance your hormones, and live a healthy lifestyle. Here, we need to distinguish between people who have low cholesterol and triglyceride levels due to poor health and poor liver function, compared to those who have low levels due to a low-fat diet and healthy lifestyle. Yes, there have been a few studies to show that sickly patients with low cholesterol and unhealthy lifestyles have rare problems like higher specific strokes. *This is due to chronic bad health, poor diet, and the inability to synthesize cholesterol normally.* It is certainly not due to low cholesterol per se at all.

DIET

In Japan, for centuries the average cholesterol level used to be about 150 mg/dL. This was due to their cultural preference for a low-fat diet based on rice, vegetables and seafood. Due to urban Westernization, they now eat much more red meat, poultry, eggs, and even dairy products. These foods were rarely eaten there. Now the average cholesterol level is about 180 mg/dL, and *heart and artery disease have gone up accordingly.* The Japanese now suffer from far more hypercholesterolemia, hypertension, atherosclerosis, aneurisms, strokes, and heart attacks. When 125 million people raise their average cholesterol and suffer a resultant rise in heart and artery disease, the results are clear and inarguable. The rural Japanese do not suffer such problems generally, as they have not adopted the western diet. This is especially true of the rural and older Okinawans. The traditional Japanese continue to enjoy good health.

SCIENTIFIC STUDIES

An excellent review from St. Bartholemew's Hospital in London settles this quite well. They went over ten of the largest cohort studies ever done on cholesterol. Every study agreed that *the lower the cholesterol the better,* regardless of any other factors. The authors concluded, "All of them show a similar effect, and none provide any evidence for a threshold below which there ceases to be an effect. The two largest studies provide strong evidence against a threshold over the range of serum cholesterol covered by the studies," (*Atherosclerosis* v 118, 1995).

The high cholesterol crowd loves to refer to an article in the *New England Journal of Medicine* (v 320, 1989). What the doctors really said is that taking all strokes together (hemorrhagic and non-hemorrhagic), the lower your cholesterol level the longer you'll live, *and the less total strokes you'll suffer.* A few sickly, elderly people, with low cholesterol, had slightly more hemorrhagic strokes. However, they were eating high-fat, high-sugar diets, and their bodies could no longer produce sufficient cholesterol. *Their low levels were due to pathology,* not good diet.

The MRFIT Study of 350,977 men found *the lower your total cholesterol the better.* Men with TC levels of 140 mg/dL to 159 mg/dL only had sixty cardiovascular deaths and fifteen strokes a year. Men with levels of 220 mg/dL to 239 mg/dL had a stunning five hundred sixty-two cardiovascular deaths and thirty-nine strokes. Which would be preferred, sixty deaths or five hundred sixty-two deaths?

CONCLUSION

The average American has a total cholesterol level over 240 mg/dL. People who promote this, "don't let your cholesterol get too low" propaganda, are simply trying to justify eating unhealthy high fat foods and lowering the standards of good health. This propaganda promotes that there is an increase in deaths due to diseases when the cholesterol level is less than 180 mg/dL, but a substantial portion of these deaths seemed to be due to poor health unrelated to low cholesterol.

15. Hormone Balancing

Your body produces several types of hormones and they play a role in essentially every process in our body. When your hormones are out of balance, you many experience a wide range of symptoms that can affect mood, energy level, and it may also lead to more serious conditions. In this chapter you are going to read about the influence of hormone levels on blood lipid profiles. Cholesterol is actually the primary source of all our other sex hormones. Did your doctor ever test your basic hormone levels after finding high cholesterol and/or triglycerides? In fact, did your doctor ever suggest testing your basic hormone levels for any reason? Even endocrinologists have no idea that your basic hormones affect blood fat levels. The main thing to understand about our hormones is that *they all work together harmoniously in concert as a team.* Therefore, we need to balance all of the main hormones as much as possible. When one hormone is deficient (or excessive) the others simply cannot function properly. We are going to talk about estrogens, testosterone, T3/T4, DHEA, pregnenolone, insulin (as blood sugar response), progesterone, melatonin, cortisol, as well as the growth hormone. *Men and women have exactly the same hormones*, only in different amounts. This could be complex, giving citations for the hundreds of published studies, but our goal is to simplify it for the reader.

In 2002 the Mississippi Regional Cancer Center published a study, "Hypercholesteremia Treatment: A New Hypothesis." This excellent work showed that our general endocrine system has much control over cholesterol and triglycerides. They treated each patient individually with bioidentical DHEA, testosterone, pregnenolone, estrogens, progesterone, and cortisol. They normalized blood fats by balancing the hormone levels of their patients with natural hormone replacement therapy. This is unique, professional, and thorough science. It is doctors like this that will lead us into the age of medical enlightenment. A stunning study!

ESTROGEN

It is a sacred myth in our society that women are somehow "deficient" in estrogen after menopause, and need estrogen supplementation. The truth is that both men and women over fifty, especially in the developed countries, are generally excessive in both estradiol and estrone. This is due to many factors such as dietary fat intake, obesity, excessive caloric intake, lack of exercise, and alcohol consumption. One in eight American women will end up with breast cancer. Research shows this is a direct effect of high estrogen (estradiol and estrone) levels. One in three women will end up with a hysterectomy, which is also a direct effect of excessive estrogen. The current program of routine estrogen supplementation for women is a deadly farce. Statistics show that three-fourths of American men, by age seventy-five, have prostate cancer. All of them will end up with this cancer if they live long enough. Research reveals that this, too, is a direct effect of excessive estrogen levels. Studies around the world, from institutions such as Columbia University and St. Luke's Hospital, show repeatedly that high estrogen levels in men are associated with cardiovascular disease in general. Men and women should test their free (not bound) levels of estradiol and estrone to see if they are excessive. If you are too high, you can *reduce fat intake,* lose weight, exercise, eat more fiber, and stop drinking alcohol. A study at the Pritikin Longevity Center lowered male estrogen levels (along with cholesterol and triglycerides) dramatically, in only twenty-six days, simply by giving the men a whole grain, low-fat diet, and regular exercise. Excessive estrogen levels have many other dangerous side effects in both men and women.

Medical doctors, including endocrinologists, don't have the term "estriol" in their vocabulary. Normal pharmacies don't carry it and can't order it. Estriol is the "forgotten estrogen," even though it comprises 80 to 90 per cent of total estrogen in both men and women.

Dosage: You can take proven supplements like 200 mg of di-indolyl methane (DIM) and 1 to 2 grams of flax oil. Women should test their estriol levels with a saliva kit. If low, use a transdermal cream or gel, or sublingual estriol, but never oral estriol salts. Men do not need to test for this.

TESTOSTERONE

Both men and women should test their testosterone levels for many reasons. Women may be normal, deficient, or excessive in testosterone. Men can only be normal or deficient. Men cannot have hyper levels even if they take supplements. Testosterone deficiency is a very important influence in heart and circulatory disease. Men have about ten times more testosterone in their blood than women do. If a woman is excessive, she can only lower testosterone levels by diet and life style changes. There are no Magic Supplements to lower it.

Dosage: Men and women with low testosterone levels can use natural prescription testosterone gels or creams, never oral testosterone. Sublingual salts (like enanthate) work well, as natural (unsalted) testosterone tastes terrible. Men who are low need about 3 mg daily (4 mg of enanthate sublingually), and women about 150 mcg (200 mcg of enanthate sublingually) in their blood. Never use testosterone unless you have tested your-self, and proven to be deficient. The ideal is a youthful level as you had at, say, the age of thirty.

DHEA

DHEA falls generally, in both men and women, over the age of forty, and it is a vital hormone for heart and circulatory health. Women can be excessive, while men are rarely excessive. If you are too high, only diet and life style changes will lower your lev-els. There are, again, no Magic Supplements to help you do this. DHEA is known as the "life extension hormone" for good rea-son. Thousands of clinical studies have been done worldwide.

At the University of California, in San Diego, an excellent study concluded DHEA concentration is independently and inversely related to death, from any cause, and death from car-diovascular disease in men over fifty. There are many benefits to keeping a youthful DHEA level throughout life. At Saga Medical School, in Japan, they found that higher levels of DHEA are related to the favorable lipid and lipoprotein levels in men. What about women? At Medical University Hospital in Ger-many the doctors found treatment with DHEA raised the ini-tially low serum concentrations of DHEA, testosterone, and androstenedione into the normal range. Serum concentrations of SHBG and total cholesterol decreased significantly. At Gifu University, in Japan, they discovered a favorable effect of DHEA on the lipid profile of Japanese postmenopausal women.

Dosage: Never use DHEA unless you have tested your levels with either blood or saliva to prove you are low. Men have about twice as much DHEA as women, so women with low levels can try 12.5 mg (half tablets) of DHEA, and men 25 mg daily.

PROGESTERONE

Progesterone is thought of as a female hormone, but it is impor-tant for men, too. Progesterone is important for the metabolism of cholesterol. Never use synthetic prescription progestins, as they have many negative side effects, and none of the benefits of real progesterone. Progesterone is the natural antagonist to excessive estrogen levels, and is very safe and very non-toxic. Many men over fifty actually have higher estradiol and estrone levels than their post-menopausal wives! Many books have been written on the value of progesterone by such authors as John Lee.

Dosage: Use natural USP transdermal progesterone with 800 mg to 1000 mg per two ounce jar. Do not use oral progesterone, as it is not absorbed well at all. Both premenopausal women and post-menopausal women may well benefit from using transdermal natural progesterone. They will use one-half teaspoon per their monthly cycle or any two weeks of the month after menopause. Men over fifty can use a mere one-eighth teaspoon five days of the week.

PREGNENOLONE

Naturally occurring pregnenolone plays a vital part in hormone production. It is the grandmother hormone, from which our other sex hormones are derived. *This is the major memory, cognition, and brain hormone.* Pregnenolone falls quite a bit, after the age of forty, in both men and women, and then stabilizes. Saliva tests are just not available in 2012. See a doctor for a blood draw or find an Internet clinic that doesn't require one. Very little is known about the effects of pregnenolone on our blood lipids, but *it is critical to balance all our hormones together.* Youthful levels are vital to overall hormone balance. Pregnenolone replacement will become much more common as more studies are done, and more is known about it. Common sense and logic tell you to keep your pregnenolone at youthful levels throughout life, since it is an integral part of your endocrine system.

Dosage: Pregnenolone is very important to use to avoid senility, memory loss and Alzheimer's as we age. Take 100 mg of phosphatidyl serine (PS), and 500 mg of acetyl-L-carnitine (ALC) for even better results. Over the age of forty, dosages of 25 mg a day for women, and 50 mg a day for men would be reasonable.

MELATONIN

Melatonin is a powerful and miraculous hormone. We are only beginning to understand just how vital it is for our health, well being, and longevity. It is an important anti-aging hormone, and decreases from the time we are teenagers, until it almost disappears by the time we reach the age of eighty. Only recently have studies come to light showing melatonin is vital in the metabolism of cholesterol and triglycerides. This fact is unknown either to the medical profession or the general public. Studies from the University of Tokyo, University of Seville, Al-Azhar University (Egypt), and Hong Kong Polytechnic University show how vital melatonin is to cholesterol metabolism. They found melatonin induced a marked protection in terms of decreasing serum cholesterol, LDL, and triglycerides, while increasing HDL over 50 percent. Melatonin, which is secreted by the pineal gland, is the most important anti-aging hormonal factor we know of. This is a very safe and very non-toxic hormone, and a vital part of your supplement program for many, many reasons. Read one of the many books that have been written about it for more information.

Dosage: Test your melatonin level at 3:00 AM by itself with saliva, as melatonin is highest at night when we sleep. If you are over forty, men should take 3 mg, and women 1.5 mg (half tabs). *Take this only at night,* and never during the day.

T3 AND T4

Thyroid metabolism is most important for healthy cholesterol levels. You must test your free T3 and free T4, and not your TSH or T3 uptake. Hypothyroidism is epidemic in Westerners over forty. *Look for midrange levels, and do not accept low normal ones.* Synthroid (L-thyroxine) and Cytomel (triiodothyronine) are bioidentical to our own thyroid hormones. Do not let the doctors butcher or irradiate your thyroid gland. The best study was from University Hospital in Venezuala, where they found 10 percent of patients with hyperlipidemia were hypothyroid. A review from the University of Nebraska found T4 replacement therapy effectively lowers total cholesterol levels.

Dosage: If your T3 or T4 level is too high, only diet and life style will lower it. You can get inexpensive thyroid blood testing on websites like www.healthcheckusa.com without a doctor. Saliva testing will be available in the near future.

INSULIN LEVELS

Blood sugar dysmetabolism, especially diabetes, is closely related to blood lipid conditions. Hyperlipidemia is a hallmark of the metabolic syndrome. *Your fasting blood sugar should be 85 or less.* Your doctor will tell you 100 or less is "fine," but it isn't. Your fasting blood glucose must be *85 or less.* Intake of simple sugars, even honey and maple syrup, is the basic cause of excessive fasting blood glucose levels. Also, just one daily dose of caffeine (coffee, energy drinks, guarana, etc.) will also raise blood sugar severely. Caffeine is a poison to be avoided even in small amounts. It is the most popular psychoactive drug in the world.

Dosage: Insulin levels per se do not need to be tested, but rather insulin resistance. This is done with a glucose tolerance, or GTT. You drink a cup of glucose solution and wait one hour to get your blood glucose measured. Look for results at least 10 points below what the doctor will tell you is good. This reveals how well your insulin responds. Poor response is called "insulin resistance."

HUMAN GROWTH HORMONE

The Human Growth hormone is also an important factor in blood fat levels, and growth hormone falls steeply as we age. It is very difficult to get a four sample panel (at 9/1/5/9) over twelve hours. Go by real world results, instead, if you are over fifty. Testing IGF-1 levels does *not* work. If you are over the age of fifty you can bet your HGH level is low. HGH is very over-rated because it is expensive. It is expensive because it is very difficult to synthesize. Only real, prescription rhGH (recombinant human growth hormone) works. Research shows all the non-prescription supplements out there claiming to raise growth hormone (no matter how well advertised) are useless. *Life style* keeps your growth hormone level high. Do not even think of using HGH until all your other basic hormones (eleven in men and fourteen in women) are tested and balanced. *This is the very last hormone to work on.* HGH is the most overrated of all our hormones. It is a vanity more than anything.

Dosage: Exercising, staying slim, eating less, eating well, fasting regularly, not drinking or smoking, and healthy living generally all work. Injecting 1 IU daily can easily cost you three-hundred dollars a month, or three-thousand six-hundred dollars a year. The research on using rhGH in the elderly does show improvements in lowering cholesterol and triglycerides levels, as well as raising HDL and lowering LDL.

CORTISOL

We must mention cortisol (also known as hydrocortisone), the "stress hormone." There is very little information available on supplementing or lowering cortisol, and it's relation to blood lipids. The Western Infirmary in Scotland proved that healthy cortisol levels are integral to cholesterol metabolism in both men and women. High cortisol levels are epidemic in Western societies, due to stress, poor diet, and negative life style factors. You can only lower cortisol levels by better food choices, exercise, supplements, general hormone balance, and positive life style changes. You really don't need to bother with cortisol at all.

Dosage: A few people are deficient in cortisol, due to adrenal exhaustion, and may benefit from low dose oral Cortef® therapy. You need to do a four sample comprehensive saliva test (at 9/1/5/9) over twelve hours to see the daily fluctuations.

CONCLUSION

The hormones covered throughout this chapter are all vital in order for your body to function properly. Each of the basic hormones provides significant health benefits. When these hormones are imbalanced they may affect our blood lipids and cholesterol levels. Remember to regularly test your hormone levels so that you can maintain a healthy hormone balance. In the next chapter we will learn how to test our hormones without a doctor.

16. Home Hormone Testing

In the last chapter, you saw how critical hormone balance is for your blood lipid levels. Have you ever had a doctor suggest you test your hormone levels for ANY condition? Medical doctors almost never test their patients for basic hormone levels, regardless of their condition. In fact, most doctors, including New Age doctors, holistic practitioners, naturopaths, gynecologists, and life extension specialists, are simply unaware of which hormones to test, how to test them, and how to administer supplemental ones. Even endocrinologists are surprisingly uninformed about hormone testing and administration, though this is their specialty. If you were to request a hormone test from your doctor, it would require getting blood drawn, paying up to one-hundred dollars per hormone tested, going on a second office visit, and then the purchase of an expensive prescription. Don't waste your money on testing bound levels (unavailable levels) of sex hormones that tell you almost nothing. Proteins in our bloodstream called SHBG (sex hormone binding globulins) attach themselves to most of our sex hormones, making them biologically unavailable. For example, testosterone is usually about 98 percent bound, with about 2 percent free (usable) testosterone that actually affects our biological processes. L-thyroxine (T4) is also about 98 percent bound, and only about 2 percent biologically available. Therefore, it is left up to you to test your hormone levels and maintain a healthy balance.

TESTING SALIVA AND BLOOD SAMPLES

For over twenty years now, researchers in clinics have been able to accurately measure hormone levels using saliva samples rather than blood. This was often used in Third World countries, and in the field, due to the lack of available refrigeration for blood samples. The World Health Organization approved this method in the 1990's due to its practicality, accuracy, reliability, and low cost. Finally, in the late 1990's, this became available to the general public. You can now buy saliva test kits for estradiol, estrone, estriol, testosterone, androstenedione, DHEA, cortisol, melatonin, among others. California and New York have banned this, due to pressure from the medical profession. If you live in these states, simply use a return address for a friend or relative in another state. There are now Internet sites offering real blood testing without a doctor. You do not have to see a doctor to test your insulin, pregnenolone, thyroid hormones (T3 and T4), or progesterone (cannot be saliva tested as it is fat soluble). At sites like www.walkinlab.com and www.healthcheckusa.com, you can get real blood tests for these without a doctor at a cooperating clinic. Just do a Google search for, "hormone testing."

Saliva testing is a tremendous technological breakthrough in both traditional and holistic medicine. However, very few people and very few doctors are even aware of it. Strangely enough, these are not even sold in pharmacies, health food stores, or drug stores. The only place to buy saliva hormone test kits is the Internet. Again, this is due to pressure from the medical profession. No matter what your health status, *you should know your basic hormone levels*. Raise those which are low, and lower those which are excessive. Keeping youthful levels of testosterone, DHEA, melatonin, progesterone, pregnenolone, T3/T4, and GH will add years to your life, and life to your years. Even many life extension advocates, that promote the use of these hormones, don't understand that you must test your levels before using them, or the correct way to administer them. Almost no one knows what their basic hormone levels are, so they will never enjoy optimal health and lifespan.

Search the Internet for "saliva hormone test kits," and you will find the leading clinics that sell them. Also search for online labs where no doctor is needed for blood tests. Ranges are given for sex and age. Just add high and low range, and divide by two to get midrange. Remember, you want the *youthful* levels that you had at about age thirty.

The saliva labs generally offer kits that test your hormones at about thirty dollars to fifty dollars each. Melatonin has to be ordered separately, and tested at 3:00 AM. Vegetarians and macrobiotics will have lower levels of sex hormones generally. Time of day is very important for when a sample is taken. Take your samples at the same time every morning (e.g. 9:00 AM) for consistency.

CONCLUSION

Balancing your hormone levels is an important step in maintaining a healthy body. Saliva hormone testing is one of the greatest technological advances of the last decade. It is inexpensive, accurate, and practical. Now we also have Internet blood labs where no doctor is needed. Everyone can easily test most all of their basic hormones at home, inexpensively, and without a doctor.

Seven Steps to Natural Health

The following steps are of vital importance if you want to live a long and healthy life. With these seven steps you can cure "incurable" illnesses, like cancer, diabetes, heart disease, and others, naturally without drugs, surgery, or chemotherapy. Do your best to follow every step, and note that there is also an optional eighth step that recommends prayer or meditation.

1. Maintain an American macrobiotic wholegrain-based diet. Diet is the most crucial factor in achieving good health. Diet cures disease. Everything else is secondary.

2. Take proven supplements to enhance the effects of your diet. There are only about twenty scientifically recommended supplements for those over forty, and eight for those under forty.

3. Balance your hormone levels. There are fourteen basic hormones, and you can easily (and inexpensively) measure your hormone levels from the comfort of your own home.

4. Exercise regularly, even if that only means taking a thirty-minute walk every day. Exercise is vital, and it is best to have a balanced workout of aerobics and resistance training.

5. Fast one day a week, drinking only water from dinner to dinner. Fasting is the most powerful healing method known to man. Join our monthly Young Again two-day fast—the fasting calendar is at www.youngagain,org during the last weekend of every month.

6. Do not take prescription drugs, except *temporary* antibiotics or pain medication during an emergency. (Of course, there are rare exceptions. Diabetics, for example, need to take insulin.)

7. Limit or end any bad habits such as drinking alcohol or coffee, using recreational drugs, or eating desserts. You don't have to be a saint, but you do have to be sincere.

About the Author

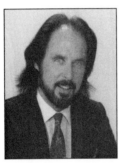

Roger Mason is an internationally known research chemist who studies natural health and longevity. He has written ten different unique and cutting edge books about his findings. He sold Beta Prostate® in 2011, walked away from radio and TV, and formed a charitable trust. He lives with his wife and dog in Wilmington, NC, where they run Young Again Products. You can get his free weekly newsletter, read his books, and his three-hundred articles for free at www.youngagain.org.

Index

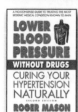

LOWER BLOOD PRESSURE WITHOUT DRUGS,
SECOND EDITION
Roger Mason

Over sixty-five million Americans have high blood pressure. Although prescription drugs may effectively treat this problem, they have potentially dangerous side effects. Fortunately, natural alternatives are available. In this updated edition of *Lower Blood Pressure Without Drugs,* best-selling author Roger Mason provides a proven nutritional approach to lowering blood pressure safely and naturally.

The book begins by explaining what hypertension is, what causes it, and how it is diagnosed. From there, it goes on to describe how a simple diet, rich in whole grains and low in fat, can improve both blood pressure and general health. This is followed by chapters that address such key topics as the best nutritional supplements to take; which exercises are most effective; how to maintain hormonal balance; and, just as important, how to overcome poor dietary and lifestyle habits. *Lower Blood Pressure Without Drugs* can be your first step towards safely and effectively improving your health.

FEBRUARY 2012 • $9.95 US • 128 pages • 6 x 9-inch quality paperback • ISBN 978-0-7570-0366-0

THE NATURAL PROSTATE CURE, SECOND EDITION
Roger Mason

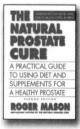

By age fifty, three out of four men have enlarged prostates, which can lead to serious health problems, and one in three men has cancer cells in his prostate. Traditional treatments for the more critical of these prostate-related illnesses include surgery, radiation, chemotherapy, and even castration. These methods are dangerous and have potentially drastic results. Worst of all, they fail to address the real cause of prostate problems.

In this updated edition of *The Natural Prostate Cure,* author Roger Mason provides a unique and effective alternative to risky prostate surgery and drug therapies. The book opens with a basic lesson in proper diet and presents the best supplements for maintaining a healthy prostate, including beta-sitosterol, a vital key to prostate well-being. The author then talks about steps that can be taken to cure prostate disease, including cancer. The last chapters of the book suggest hormone treatments that can prevent and combat these potentially serious conditions.

MARCH 2012 • $9.95 US • 128 pages • 6 x 9-inch quality paperback • ISBN 978-0-7570-0370-7

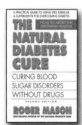

THE NATURAL DIABETES CURE, SECOND EDITION
Roger Mason

Poor nutrition is the major cause of blood sugar disorders like diabetes, but many people simply don't know how to maintain a healthy, balanced diet. For everyone who suffers from a blood sugar problem, Roger Mason is here to help with this updated edition of *The Natural Diabetes Cure.*

The Natural Diabetes Cure begins by explaining how diabetes develops, as well as its association with several severe health risks. The book then details how a balanced diet of whole grains, fresh vegetables, and healthy fats not only helps improve overall health and well-being, but also prevents conditions like high blood pressure, obesity, and insulin resistance, which can lead to type 2 diabetes. Additional chapters discuss nutritional supplements that can regulate blood sugar, and explore important topics like hormone balance and exercise. Throughout, You'll learn how you can free yourself from diabetes and enjoy a longer, higher-quality life.

MARCH 2012 • $9.95 US • 144 pages • 6 x 9-inch quality paperback • ISBN 978-0-7570-0369-1

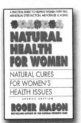

NATURAL HEALTH FOR WOMEN, SECOND EDITION
Roger Mason

Every day, millions of women go through menopause. For some, this experience includes troubling side effects such as hot flashes and depression. It may even lead to serious disorders like osteoporosis and diabetes. *Natural Health for Women* is a concise guide to coping with menopause as well as many other problems that are of concern to women.

The book first looks at menopause and explores various treatments, including hormonal therapy. The author then discusses related health issues, including osteoporosis, cardiovascular disease, diabetes, arthritis, and excess weight. Most important, he presents important information about natural foods and supplements, as well as a crucial discussion on home hormone testing.

MARCH 2012 • $9.95 US • 144 pages • 6 x 9-inch quality paperback • ISBN 978-0-7570-0368-4

TESTOSTERONE IS YOUR FRIEND, SECOND EDITION
Roger Mason

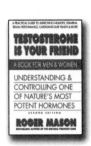

Considered the principal male sex hormone, testosterone is responsible for stimulating and controlling characteristics that are considered masculine, like muscles and hair growth. What many people don't realize is that this hormone is present to a lesser degree in females. What's more, low testosterone levels can cause countless health problems for *both* sexes, including memory loss, anxiety and depression, osteoporosis, increased cholesterol levels, weight gain, sexual dysfunction, and infertility.

In the updated edition of *Testosterone Is Your Friend*, author Roger Mason first clearly explains the important role that testosterone plays in the body. He then presents the latest and most effective natural treatments and supplements to help raise testosterone levels. You'll learn how to test your hormone levels at home and how to naturally improve not only your sex life, but every aspect of your health.

APRIL 2012 • $9.95 US • 128 pages • 6 x 9-inch quality paperback • ISBN 978-0-7570-0371-4

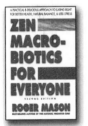

ZEN MACROBIOTICS FOR EVERYONE, SECOND EDITION
Roger Mason

In today's busy stress-filled world, making the right food choices is not always a priority. We may be considered an educated society, yet seem blind to the fact that our diets are typically unhealthy—low in whole grains, legumes, and fresh produce, and high in processed foods and sugary beverages. This places us at risk for serious health conditions, including diabetes, cardiovascular disease, and cancer. Fortunately, improving your diet is not as difficult or time-consuming as you may think.

In *Zen Macrobiotics for Everyone*, author Roger Mason expands upon the Japanese macrobiotic tradition to offer a diet that is not only wholesome but also creative, delicious, and surprisingly uncomplicated. The book begins with a concise history of the macrobiotic lifestyle. It then concentrates on simple ways in which you can incorporate macrobiotics—including the practice of meditation—in your life. Reader-friendly charts provide basic nutrition facts on the healthiest foods, making it simple to choose your foods wisely.

MAY 2012 • $9.95 US • 128 pages • 6 x 9-inch quality paperback • ISBN 978-0-7570-0372-1

**For more information about our books,
visit our website at www.squareonepublishers.com**